Talking to My Tatas

Talking to My Tatas

All You Need to Know from a
Breast Cancer Researcher and Survivor

Dana Brantley-Sieders

ROWMAN & LITTLEFIELD
Lanham • Boulder • New York • London

Published by Rowman & Littlefield
An imprint of The Rowman & Littlefield Publishing Group, Inc.
4501 Forbes Boulevard, Suite 200, Lanham, Maryland 20706
www.rowman.com

86-90 Paul Street, London EC2A 4NE

British Library Cataloguing in Publication Information Available

Library of Congress Cataloging-in-Publication Data

Names: Brantley-Sieders, Dana, author.
Title: Talking to my tatas : all you need to know from a breast cancer researcher and
   survivor / Dana Brantley-Sieders.
Description: Lanham, Maryland : Rowman & Littlefield Publishers, [2022] | Includes
   bibliographical references and index. | Summary: "Provides accessible science and health
   information for the love of your boobs, especially when they have cancer. Dana Brantley-
   Sieders spent twenty years working as a biomedical breast cancer researcher. Then, she
   was diagnosed with breast cancer. She thought she knew breast cancer before it whacked
   her upside her left boob and left her bleeding on the curb of uncertainty. Turns
   out, she had a lot to learn. This book shares Brantley-Sieders' personal journey with
   breast cancer, from the laboratory bench to her own bedside, and provides accessible
   information   about breast cancer biology for non-scientists. Talking to My Tatas: All
   You Need to Know from a Breast Cancer Researcher and Survivor, offers accurate,
   evidence-based science that is accessible to all readers,   including the more than three
   hundred thousand individuals diagnosed with breast cancer every year, their caregivers,
   and their loved ones. Knowledge is power, and lack of it can lead to overtreatment,
   unnecessary pain and suffering, and even death. By demystifying the process from
   mammograms, biopsies, pathology, and diagnostics, to surgical options, tumor genomic
   testing, and new treatment options, Brantley-Sieders aims to arm breast cancer patients
   with the tools they need to battle this disease with a healthy dose of humor, grace, and
   hope"— Provided by publisher.
Identifiers: LCCN 2021032077 (print) | LCCN 2021032078 (ebook) | ISBN
   9781538155103 (cloth) | ISBN 9781538155110 (ebook)
Subjects: LCSH: Brantley-Sieders, Dana,—Health. | Breast—Cancer—Patients—United
   States—Biography. | Breast cancer—Patients—Treatment.
Classification: LCC RC280.B8 B647 2022 (print) | LCC RC280.B8 (ebook) | DDC
   616.99/4490092 [B]--dc23
LC record available at https://lccn.loc.gov/2021032077
LC ebook record available at https://lccn.loc.gov/2021032078

~

Contents

              and Hope   201

              Appendix   216

              Notes   229

              Bibliography   252

              Index   275

              About the Author   279

Acknowledgments

Many amazing people helped me bring this book to life, including an army of health-care professionals and a community of family, friends, and survivors who've helped me not only survive my adventure with breast cancer but also thrive in the wake of it. Thank you to Drs. Patricia Tepper, Angie Larson, Ingrid Meszoely, Galen Perdikis, Brent Rexer, Melinda Sanders, and Bapsi Chak Chakravarthy and to their teams of anesthesiologists, nurses, fellows, residents, technicians, and staff. You saved my life and made me whole, and most of you have seen my boobs in all of their iterations.

In addition to saving my life, the amazing and wonderful Drs. Meszoely, Perdikis, and Rexer, along with Dr. Ben Ho Park, mentor and incredible human being, answered about a million questions (each), fact-checked and proofed chapters with clinical information, and helped me out tremendously with this project. Special thanks to Dr. Jin Chen, my mentor, longtime collaborator, and dear friend, for fact-checking chapters on tumor immunology. Any mistakes in those chapters are mine, not theirs. Thanks also to Dr. David Vaught for his comments and suggestions.

Thank you to my incredible literary agent, Barbara Collins-Rosenberg. She believed in the proposal and project and worked tirelessly to make sure it found the right home. Thank you to my wonderful editor,

Suzanne Staszak-Silva, for her guidance. She made this book shine! Thank you also to all of the amazing people at Rowman & Littlefield for bringing this book to readers—specifically, my production editor, Elaine McGarraugh, assistant editor Deni Remsberg, and copy editor Deborah F. Justice. I owe a special debt of gratitude to Alice Sullivan, who helped me craft the book proposal that shaped this book, landed my agent, and ultimately got me the book deal.

No one has your back like survivor sisters (and brothers). I owe a huge debt of gratitude to Pam Jasper, Linda Horton, Janet Piper, Tanisha Jones, Sue Daugherty Draughn, Cynthia D'Alba, Betsy Gray, Daniëlle van Zijl, Em Shotwell, Karen Pugh, Lisa Turpin Stephens, Lisa Strunk Quig, Lynn Cahoon, Mary Walters, Deb Harrison Kuhns, Lillian Boeskool, Ronei Harden-Moroney, Hollye Salazar Cross, J. C., Gerry Milligan, Paul Bushdid, and many more who have touched my life and shared their cancer stories with me. Thanks to my hero/mom, Carol McNeil Brantley, who is also a breast cancer survivor. I acknowledge and thank those in the great beyond, like my cousin—who was more like a sister—Sherri Killian and my uncle Jack Brantley, whose spirits live on in our hearts and minds. Shout-out to survivor friends in cyberspace on Facebook pages, like Breast Cancer Straight Talk and Finding Humor After Breast Cancer. These amazing people have kept me going, lifted me out of fogs and funk, talked me off ledges, and shared laughs, love, and secrets only cancer survivors know. I am forever grateful.

Shout-out to the wonderful mentors and collaborators I've been lucky enough to work with over the years in the laboratory, including Drs. Michael Torres, Terry Bunde, Robert Naylor, Lynnette Sievert, Paul Threadgill, Lynn Matrisian, Rebecca Cook, Daniel Medina, Ambra Pozzi, Pampee Young, Joey Barnett, Julie Rhoades, James Thomas, Leslie Crofford, Ann Richmond, Maureen Gannon, Mark de Caestecker, and Ben Ho Park, Craig Duvall, Jane Wu, Nikki Cheng, Wei Bin Fang, Rachelle Johnson, Shan Wang, Deanna Edwards, Justin Balko, and Gavin Bennett. These people have made me the scientist I am today, and many of them have kept me going during and after my breast cancer diagnosis. I am so grateful for you all.

I've been fortunate enough to mentor or comentor many talented and dedicated research assistants, graduate and medical students, and postdoctoral fellows over the years. These incredible physicians and scientists (or soon-to-be physicians and scientists) include Drs. Justin Caughron, Charlene Dunaway Altamirano, Krishna Sarma, David Vaught, Meghana Rao, Victoria Youngblood, Kalin Wilson, Debra Walter, Meghan Morrison-Joly, Thomas Werfel, Meredith Jackson, Samantha Sarett, Ella Hoogenboezem, Shrusti Patel, Verra Ngwa, and Eileen Shiuan. Mentorship is one of the most rewarding parts of my work in academics, and I thank each of you for the privilege and trust you put in me. Know that I'm forever proud of you.

I am grateful to my family, the people who are my reason for being and who love me unconditionally. I thank my husband, Patrick Sieders, for being my champion, best friend, and partner. When I told him I had cancer, he declared himself captain of Team Dana Beats Cancer and has been the most supportive and loving spouse. He really took that whole in-sickness-and-in-health part of the wedding vows seriously even though he got more than he bargained for. I'm a lucky woman. My children, Anastacia and Jason, the incredible people I birthed who amaze me every single day, have helped me through my battle with cancer and give me a reason to keep fighting. I love you both to the ends of the universe and back. And I cannot forget my four-legged home nurses who healed and soothed me with purrs and lots of love.

~

Introduction

I Love You with All My Boobs. I Would Say My Heart, but My Boobs Are Bigger.

Breasts, boobs, boobies, tatas, tits, titties, hooters, bazoobs, baps, fun bags, melons, knockers, chesticles, coconuts, fried eggs, milk monsters, the girls, maracas, slammers, bazoombas, breasticles, bazookas, bosoms, jubblies, twins, peaks, rack, shelf, tatty bo jangles, tatties, cans, bub-balas, bongos, bouncers, hooters, muchachas, fleshy mounds, bewbs, kahunas, golden globes, headlamps, baby buffets, shoulder boulders, honkers, chebs, zeppelins, Goodyears, beestings, molehills, lady bumps, lady lumps (thanks, Fergie), boobages, ninnies, gozongas, nei neis, bo-ingley-doinglies, jiggly puffs, colt .45s, bikini stuffers, norks, breastesses, wangers, sweater kittens, love apples, perkies, yayas, chi chis, big guns, double whammies, bombshells, gazongas, bubbies, yayas . . .

(.) (.)
(.)(.)
(.)(.)
(^) (^)
(. y .)
(. v .)
(o)(o)

1

No matter what you call them, breasts are and always have been an endless source of fascination throughout history and across cultures. They've been celebrated in paintings, sculptures, poetry, song lyrics, and porn. They are icons of femininity and symbolize the duality of womanhood and feminine identity/presentation, at least as it exists in the Judeo-Christian-Islamic traditions. Objects of lust or nurturing, female empowerment or sexual exploitation, the wanton wench versus the maternal Madonna, breasts have always been front and center. (See what I did there?)

They're used to capture the (straight, cis) male gaze in order to sell everything from cars to sodas. Men either want to see them all the time or want them covered up and restrained; breasts are essentially the perfect metaphor for what the patriarchy (stop arguing; the patriarchy is totally a thing) wants from women. But this book isn't about what *men* think of other people's breasts (sorry-not-sorry, fellas, but you've gotten way too much page time already). This book is about a person's relationship with their own breasts—specifically, my relationship with mine before, during, and after a breast cancer diagnosis. These pages are full of science, social commentary, swear words, and, ultimately, hope. As a biomedical researcher who has spent the past twenty years (and counting) researching the causes of and potential new treatments for breast cancer, I've acquired quite a bit of knowledge from the front lines of the war on cancer. As a caregiver for loved ones who've suffered from breast cancer, I've seen the horrors, heartaches, and triumphs that cancer patients experience. As a patient and survivor, I've experienced some of those things firsthand. These are some of the reasons I wrote this book.

Another reason I wrote this book is because as a pathologically enthusiastic nerd, I've made it my mission to make science more accessible to nonscientists. In general, people in my field spend inordinate amounts of time talking to one another, but we don't talk enough to the public. That's a shame, especially considering that most of us are funded by the National Institutes of Health through the National Cancer Institute and by the Department of Defense Breast Cancer Research Program, which are, in turn, funded by tax dollars. As such, I personally believe that I should be able to explain my research to anyone in terms they can understand and justify why what I'm doing is important. This is especially true today.

At the time of this writing—late 2020, early 2021—a pervasive and insidious antiscience movement has gripped the United States and the wider world. While cancer researchers aren't battling the same suppressive forces as climate scientists or those fighting COVID-19, our endeavors and findings are still often met with a lack of interest, a lack of understanding, skepticism, and hostility from a small but vocal segment of the population. Some are convinced that we are incompetent— *Why, after all of this time and money, haven't you cured cancer?* Others think we're a part of some conspiracy—that we've already found the cure for cancer and are suppressing it, hiding it from the public so we can continue to profit from some sort of Cancer-Industrial Complex. We're apparently like the Illuminati, only not as stylish or popular.

I've been called a pharma shill even though I've never been personally funded by the pharmaceutical industry. I even had one charming individual on Facebook tell me he hoped I would get chemo as punishment for denying the "truth" that cannabis cures cancer.

Spoiler alert: It doesn't. (More on that in chapter 10.)

I also wanted to share my story because of my unique perspective. As a breast cancer researcher, I thought I knew breast cancer. I had lost loved ones and watched others endure surgery, chemotherapy, radiation, and hormone-suppression therapy, including a close cousin, my own mother, and one of my closest friends. But I learned that there's a big difference between watching it and living it, and when I heard the words, "You have cancer," in my doctor's office on April 19, 2018, I was as terrified, frozen, and unprepared as every other person faced with those three terrible, life-changing words. While going through diagnostic tests, surgery prep, four surgeries and counting, radiation, and postradiation treatments, my two lives as a breast cancer research scientist and a breast cancer patient collided, and I emerged with a new purpose.

Well, not immediately. It's not like I woke up covered in pink ribbon–embossed armor, wielding the sword of the cancer warrior and the shield of bodacious tatas. First I needed a few years to get the tumors cut out (including the primary tumors and residual disease we found later), come to terms with my Frankenboobs—perky, but covered in gnarly keloid scars (only the right one, though, because the left got zapped with radiation, which is really good for scarring but terrible for texture and sensation; see chapter 16 for more on my reconstruction surgeries)—start and stop three estrogen blockers until I found one I could tolerate (the first two were terrible), and get busy getting on with life. I spent a lot of time worrying, fretting, being lost in my own head, and working myself to a near breakdown to avoid thinking about and dealing with the emotional devastation of my disease. *Is it really gone? What if it comes back? How long do I have to feel old and worn-out from fatigue, joint and muscle pain, and hot flashes? Ten years of antiestrogen therapy? That's a prison term! Why hasn't anyone come up with something to relieve hot flashes, sexual dysfunction, and all of the other indignities that come with this disease?*

These are questions I still struggle with today. So why should you listen to me, a certified lab rat sheltered in the ivory tower of academia who seems to have more questions than answers? For starters, I do have some answers and quite a bit of information that can help you if you should become part of the One in Eight Women Who Gets Breast Cancer Club.[1] (We should really get jackets and free drinks for life.) After working in the laboratory with breast cancer cells in a culture dish—which are then transplanted into animal models and used to extract and analyze the DNA, RNA, and proteins to find the changes that make once-normal cells go rogue (don't worry—I'll define all of these terms) and to find out how we can target those changes to kill cancer cells—I've learned quite a bit about what makes cancer tick at the molecular, genetic, and cellular levels. Cancer's mission is simple: grow and survive. Cancer rewrites the fundamental rules that govern the function of cells in your body. Cells are supposed to work for the good of the collective—the host, you. They keep you alive, defend you against invading diseases, heal and repair damage, and work in harmony to keep the machine that is your body working properly to carry you through life.

When normal cells transform into cancer cells, they stop caring about the good of the collective—the host. Cancer cells highjack resources and systems in your body for themselves, taking your nutrients to sustain their own malignant growth by tricking your body into sending a blood supply, hiding from your immune system, and, more often than not, tricking your immune system into working to help the cancerous cells thrive. They do this by altering the cells and scaffolding around the bundle of cancer cells and cells from the microenvironment to form a tumor mass that gives the cancer cells shelter and the means to travel to other parts of your body. (We'll cover that in chapters 2 and 16.)

And cancer cells do much of this before you even know they're there. Cancer is sneaky. Cancer is insidious. Cancer is relentless.

Wait, scratch that—*cancers are* relentless. Cancer isn't a single disease—even breast cancers. They are actually a collection of related diseases that are as unique as the human beings in which they grow. That's one of the reasons why cancers are so difficult to treat and why we haven't cured "the cancer" yet. "The cancer" doesn't exit. (More on that later.)

But cancers aren't invincible. They can be detected earlier and earlier, thanks to advances in diagnostics. There are drugs that can more precisely seek out and destroy cancer cells while minimizing harm to normal tissue. More recently, drugs that harness the power of the immune system and emerging anticancer vaccines have shown unprecedented success for killing some cancers. Ongoing research aims to expand antitumor immunity to more and more cancers. Are these cures? That's a tricky question. Remember, cancers are sneaky. You can show *no evidence of disease* (NED) for months, years, and even decades before the cancer cells hiding in your body wake up and wreak havoc.

> *Note:* you can also live a full and healthy life span with NED, which is what we want for every cancer patient; or, if not NED, then we want cancer patients to live a relatively normal, healthy life span in spite of their tumor burden, by keeping the tumor controlled or in a state of dormancy.

Some of the most important questions in cancer research relate to dormancy: *What keeps leftover cancer cells in a resting state*, and, perhaps more importantly, *What wakes them up?* I'll tackle all of this and more in part 1 of this book, and in part 3 I'll provide a crash course on scientific literacy. This part will teach you how to separate fact from pseudoscience scams and also teach you how to look past sensational headlines to discover what scientific studies actually do (and don't) show. I don't have all of the answers, but I can share hopeful news about better survival rates, the latest research, and what's on the horizon.

Through sharing my story, I can offer assurance to patients and survivors that they are not alone.

That gets to what I write about in part 2 of my book—my own bout with breast cancer, where I'll let you in on the very human side of breast cancer. These chapters were the most difficult to write, like ripping the bandage off a raw and gaping wound and exposing the dark ugliness and unexpected beauty of the healing process for all to see. Being a scientists and knowing cancer on an intellectual level is one thing; experiencing cancer on a deep, personal, and visceral level challenged me in a way I'd never been challenged before. It threw me up against a wall and asked, "What are you made of?"

Survivors and those embarking on their own battle with cancer understand this all too well, but we also learn about a secret weapon that cancer cannot bend or break: We have each other. We are many, we are tough, and we are strong, but we are also allowed to fall into the arms of all the other survivors out there who've been through it when our strength wanes. We can lift one another up, make each other laugh, and, somehow, make it through this journey we never asked to take. I'll cover that in part 4 of this book. I'm not the only cancer researcher to battle cancer, but I'm the only one who can tell this particular story—my story. I hope it makes you laugh. I hope it makes you think. I'm sorry if it makes you cry. But, ultimately, I hope it gives you hope.

> *Quick note:* Don't skip out on the chapter notes provided at the end of the book. I've included additional information there, along with resources for further reading and the occasional snarky comments that I hope will give you a chuckle.

~

PART I

BREAST BIOLOGY, BREAST CANCER, AND WHAT TO EXPECT WITH A BREAST CANCER DIAGNOSIS

~

CHAPTER ONE

Can I Talk to You about My Personal Relationship with My Breasts?

Breasts, in addition to being symbols of femininity, beauty, and desire, are incredible organs in terms of development, structure, and function. Much of what we know about how the mammary-glandular epithelium—which makes up the internal network of ducts that connect milk-producing acini (small sac-like cavities in a gland that are surrounded by secretory cells) at the end of the ducts to the nipple—comes from studying mice.[1] (See further below for more details about animal research and why it is necessary.)

Mice obviously aren't people, and there are some pretty significant differences in terms of numbers of glands (mice have five pairs of mammary glands, whereas humans have two breasts), hormonal-regulation context (mice have an estrous cycle, whereas humans have a menstrual cycle), and structural and anatomical features (mice have a single lactiferous duct connecting the glandular epithelial network to the nipple, whereas multiple lactiferous ducts connect to the nipple in humans). Yet for all of these differences and the evolutionary gap between mice and people, the embryonic development of mammary glands, growth during puberty, and cyclic remodeling during and after each round of pregnancy are remarkably similar. Rodents also serve as excellent models for understanding malignant transformation in mammary epithelium, the process that leads to cancer.[2] The American

Association for Cancer Research has a video that provides an excellent overview of how mouse models have revolutionized our understanding of cancer and how to treat it.[3] So, starting with that framework, let's delve a little into some cool science with the basics of mammary-gland anatomy, structure, and function. Don't worry—there'll be no test and no judgement. This is a judgement-free book, y'all, and I'll make sure the science is accessible, easy to understand, and, above all else, fun. I'm just that kind of girl—a pathologically enthusiastic nerd. It's important to understand normal physiology and function as a context for understanding how things get messed up in cancer. My own research is focused on understanding normal mammary-gland growth and development at the molecular level and using that knowledge as a framework for understanding how these processes go awry when normal tissue transforms into cancer.

Mammary-Gland Anatomy, Structure, and Function

Anyone who owns breasts, no matter how big or how small, or anyone who has played with them can appreciate how wonderfully bouncy and squishy breasts are—so comfortable and comforting. That's mostly due to fat, the adipose tissue that cushions the milk-producing and -delivering glandular epithelium, specialized cells that make up alveoli (the milk-producing mammary epithelium) and ducts (the network of tubes through which milk travels to the nipple to feed nursing babies). These structures are depicted in the left panel of figure 1.1. The left panel shows an artistic rendering of a human breast. The squishy, bouncy fat provides support for the networks of epithelial ducts that end in grape-like clusters of milk-making glands. The grape-like clusters are connected by milk-shuttling ducts that lead to the nipple, which delivers milk to nursing babies. The right panels show whole-mount preparations of mammary glands from a mouse, which is just a fancy way of saying we took pieces of breast tissue, squished them on slides, stained them so we can actually see the glands that are embedded in the fat of mammary glands from mice. The shape and structure of mouse mammary glands are strikingly similar to human tissue. This makes mice a good model for breast cancer research.

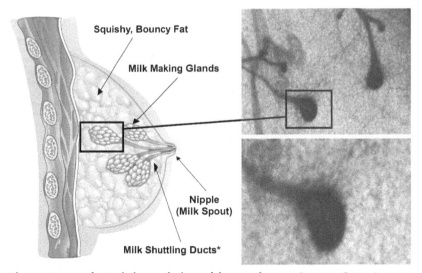

Squishy, Bouncy Fat

Milk Making Glands

Nipple
(Milk Spout)

Milk Shuttling Ducts*

Figure 1.1. *Left:* Artistic rendering of human breast. *Source:* Getty Images. *Right:* Breast and mammary-gland anatomy. *Source:* Dana M. Brantley-Sieders, whole-mount images of mouse mammary-gland preparation.

Note: Most breast cancers originate from cells in the duct.

There are other specialized cell types, including myoepithelial cells, which contain contractile fibers similar to muscle. These cells surround ducts and help push milk from alveoli to the nipple. While around 10 to 15 percent of invasive breast cancers arise from alveolar cells (lobular carcinoma), the majority of invasive breast cancers in humans, approximately 80 percent, come from ductal epithelial cells (ductal carcinoma). Connective tissue rich in collagen surrounds the milk-producing cells, providing structural support and anchoring the tubular glands in place.

Figure 1.2 shows the cycle of mammary-gland growth and development into a milk-production and -delivery factory during pregnancy and lactation. The network of milk-making and milk-shuttling epithelial structures exists in a resting state for most of the owner's life, just chillin', only gearing up for milk making and milk delivery during pregnancy, when the baby is on board, and after the birth of the baby, when

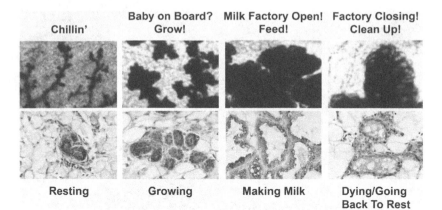

| Chillin' | Baby on Board?
Grow! | Milk Factory Open!
Feed! | Factory Closing!
Clean Up! |
| Resting | Growing | Making Milk | Dying/Going
Back To Rest |

Figure 1.2. Mammary-gland cycle. *Source:* Dana M. Brantley-Sieders, whole-mount images of mouse mammary-gland preparations and images of tissue sections from mouse mammary glands. Dana M. Brantley, Fiona E. Yull, Rebecca S. Muraoka, Donna J. Hicks, Christopher M. Cook, and Lawrence D. Kerr, "Dynamic Expression and Activity of NF-kappaB during Post-natal Mammary Gland Morphogenesis," *Mechanisms of Development* 97, nos. 1–2 (October 2000): 149–55, https://doi.org/10.1016/S0925-4773(00)00405-6.

the milk factory is open to feed it. During pregnancy, alveolar epithelial cells (which resemble broccoli florets) at the ends of the ductal stalks multiply and start making milk proteins and fats that they then deposit into central collecting lumens. When the offspring nurses, suction and the contraction of myoepithelial cells (specialized cells that surround the ducts and, like muscles, squeeze) move milk from the holding tanks of the lumen down the ductal tubes to the nipple and then to the hungry mouth of the offspring. When the offspring stops nursing, it's time for the factory to close. Most of the milk-producing alveolar cells die, returning the mammary gland to its resting state—similar to the resting state before pregnancy. The mammary gland goes through this cycle during each pregnancy, making it one of the most actively remodeling tissues in the mammalian body. The top panels in figure 1.2 show whole-mount preparations, and the lower panels show thin slices, or sections, through the tissue, processed and stained to show the architecture of the gland in cross section.

My Personal Relationship with My Breasts

In the next chapter, I'll cover how normal mammary epithelial cells, mostly the milk-shuttling ductal cells, transform into cancer cells. I'll also talk about how cancers progress from confined masses of uncontrollably growing cells to invading nightmares that spread locally to lymph nodes and systemically to other organs, including the liver, lungs, bones, and brain, through a process called metastasis.

But first, it's story time.

Long before I became a scientist, studying the ins and outs of the marvelous mammary gland and breast cancer, I was a little girl who wanted to grow up and have my very own big, bouncy breasts. I remember when the girls in my class started developing their breasts, and I was so excited to get mine.

I had also recently discovered the wonders of dirty magazines by way of an old *Adam and Eve* catalog under the cushions of my parents' couch downstairs. My next-door neighbor and I spent hours mulling over photos of (very hairy) nude and seminude men and women, wondering what exactly a vibrator was. It was a new, exciting, mysterious world just waiting to be discovered, where voluptuous women and chiseled men played forbidden games that were barely out of reach but that promised to us, someday, a set of full, perky breasts upon admission.

While boys get wider shoulders and muscles and pop boners, those signs of manly manhood on the horizon don't have the same cultural significance as breasts. There's just something magical about boobs. I mean, I'm a cis-hetero female, and I definitely appreciate a nice rack, as do many of my gay male friends. They're soft, round, and inviting. They make for awesome squishy hugs, and let's not forget their function. They feed babies, y'all.

We literally have built-in vending machines for the tiny humans that we push out of our bodies.

Mammals are the best!

No offense to birds, fish, reptiles, amphibians, or arthropods, but, seriously—fur, hair, a neocortex, and milk are some kickass evolutionary advances. (Fist bump to marsupials.)

Eventually, of course, I got my breasts, and most everything was great. Until it wasn't. I've endured multiple biopsies, surgeries to remove

cancer and reconstruct my breasts, radiation therapy, medically induced menopause, and all of the physical, mental, and emotional
fallout that comes along with it. I am not done with cancer; I'm living
with it. I may have no evidence of disease, but for my type of breast
cancer, recurrence (i.e., when the cancer comes back) in another part
of my body can crop up years or decades later. That's the harsh reality.

But having breasts totally became okay again for me. Cancer does
not consume me as a human being. It does not own me. I live with
gratitude and hope, and I will continue to fight this disease inside my
laboratory and in the public sphere. That's how, no matter my eventual
outcome, I'll ultimately win. If you have cancer or are a survivor, you'll
win too. You *are* winning. You are survivors. My hope is to arm you
with the knowledge to empower you in your fight. So, let's get started.

Why Do Scientists Have to Use Research Animals for Their Studies?

The use of whole, living animals as model systems for scientific and
disease research—referred to as *in vivo* models—is one of the most
maligned and misunderstood aspects of biological research. Animals
are cute. They are also living, breathing creatures that feel pain and
distress in ways that are all too relatable for human beings. Organizations focused on animal rights have agendas that range from seeking
to ensure that we treat animals (domestic livestock, pets, research
animals, and wildlife) ethically to working to destroy entire industries
based on the use and consumption of animals. As a scientist with over
twenty years of experience in laboratory research that involves mouse
models, I want to take the opportunity to explain why we still need to
use animal models and how we perform animal experiments ethically,
using cancer as an example.

Cancer starts out in one location in the patient's body—for example, the breast. This is called a *primary tumor*. In order for the cancer
to grow and survive, it needs to acquire nutrition and oxygen from the
body and surrounding normal tissue, referred to as the *host*. As I'll cover
in later chapters, cancer can and often does spread to other parts of the
body. It does this by a series of complex interactions with host tissue
that involve invading surrounding tissue by moving around other cells

and extracellular connective tissue and ultimately into blood vessels or lymph nodes. Some tumor cells travel through circulation, manage to somehow avoid the immune system, exit circulation, and colonize a different organ. This is called a secondary tumor, or *metastasis*. More often than not, there are multiple secondary tumors—*metastases*—some of which are detectable by imaging and some of which are not yet detectable—*micrometastases*.

That's a lot of steps involving not only the cancer cells but also blood vessels, the circulatory and the lymphatic systems, the immune system, and other distant organs colonized by cells from the primary tumor to form metastases. It is impossible to replicate these complex interactions and processes outside of a whole, living *organism* (i.e., living thing); and for breast cancer, that living organism needs to be a mammal, possessing the glandular cells required to produce and deliver milk, with the fat, blood vessels, lymph nodes, and structural-support tissue.

That being said, we as scientists go through rigorous training to make sure we use animal models appropriately, and our animal research studies are regulated in the United States by the Office of Laboratory Animal Welfare (OLAW), which is within the National Institutes of Health (NIH), the major source of funding for academic disease research, of which the National Cancer Institute that funds academic cancer disease research is a part.[4] If we do not follow federal laws and guidelines for performing animal experiments and caring for the well-being of our laboratory animals, we can lose funding, face fines, and be prosecuted under federal law. We also care for our laboratory animals because it is the right thing to do—and because failing to do so would compromise the validity of our scientific data, which could have dire consequences on how we translate those findings to the clinic for treatment of human cancer patients.

Before we even think about performing an animal experiment, we are required by law and by our academic organizations' Institutional Animal Care and Use Committees (IACUC) to submit a detailed plan for the studies.[5] These animal protocols cover issues including (1) the number of animals we propose to use in our studies, always with the goal of reducing the number of animals proposed by rigorous testing in nonanimal models and by statistical calculations of the minimum number of animals required to detect significant changes in our endpoints (e.g., tumor size, number of metastases, etc.), (2) a scientific and ethical justification for why the research is necessary that is clear to lay persons and that includes an explanation for how humans will benefit from the research we propose, (3) why it is necessary to use the specific animal model we propose and why these models cannot be replaced by nonanimal models, (4) details about the experiments (disease induction, genetic modification, testing experimental therapeutics, and so on) and how the animals will be monitored before, during, and after each procedure to reduce the risk of more than momentary pain and suffering, (5) what we will do to relieve the animals' pain and distress that might result from our experiments, and (6) humane end points (i.e., what conditions would result in termination of the experiment and euthanasia to end the animals' pain and suffering).

It's a lot. I've written several of these protocols in meticulous detail. The IACUC committees (made up of peer scientists, veterinarians, and often stakeholders) review the protocol submitted by the lead scientist—or principal investigator (PI)—and make suggestions for changes to address the welfare of the animals to maintain compliance with federal law, before sending it back to the PI. The PI then addresses the concerns by revising the protocol. Once approved, the protocol must be followed, and laboratories are subject to both IACUC and OLAW inspection to make sure we're following all protocols and the rules. Many institutions seek and maintain accreditation by the American Association for Laboratory Animal Science (AALAS).[6] The animals are housed in specialized facilities monitored by trained veterinarians and technicians: they are fed, watered, given enrichment to ensure their psychological well-being, and treated for any issues arising from experimental manipulation or illnesses not related to research.

Again, noncompliance can result in fines, further inspections, or loss of animal-experimentation privileges for the individual laboratory up to the academic institution as a whole. It's a *big* deal. We do not take our responsibilities lightly, and, unlike the cosmetic industry, the work we do with animals has and will continue to lead to knowledge about and new treatments for human disease and will improve the lives of people and the condition of humanity.[7]

CHAPTER TWO

~

Cancer 101

What (Breast) Cancer Is and
How It Makes Your Body Betray You

This is a crash course. There are many books solely devoted to the bio-logical processes that lead to cancer development and disease progres-sion. I recommend *The Emperor of All Maladies: A Biography of Cancer* by Dr. Siddhartha Mukherjee, an oncologist and born storyteller who covers the topic in great detail.[1] His book includes the history of the diseases, from diagnosis to treatment to political movements leading to the creation of the Congressionally Directed Medical Research Programs (CDMRP) under the Department of Defense (DOD), which started with breast cancer research support and now funds research aimed at discovering better treatments for a wide array of human diseases.[2] I mention DOD CDMRP specifically because it was my first source of funding as a graduate student when I started working in the field of breast cancer and has supported my research endeavors ever since, along with the National Cancer Institute. For a deep dive into the general topic of cancer, grab Dr. Mukherjee's book.

This chapter covers the basics in broad strokes.

The Molecular-Genetic Basis of Cancer

Cancer has been with us since we became human—even before.[3] It's poetic, in a really twisted, fucked up way, since cancer *is* us. Cancer

17

was once healthy tissue, starting out as a cell in your body, fulfilling its duty to keep the collective whole—you—functioning. This cell toed the line, divided when it was supposed to, stopped dividing when it was supposed to, differentiated—or specialized—to perform its function, and if it had remained normal, it might have died when told to do so after that function was fulfilled. Which brings us to three of the hallmarks of cancer: uncontrolled cell division, failure to respond to the normal programs that put the brakes on cell division, and failure to undergo programmed cell death. These malfunctions are part of what transforms a cell from normal to malignant—or cancerous. There are more cancer hallmarks,[4] which I will touch on in later chapters, but these are the fundamentals.[5]

The question for scientists and health-care providers is . . . *How?* How does cancer form? How does it survive? How does it die? The *why* is sort of wrapped up in the how, but, honestly, we're less interested in the deeper philosophical meaning and existential implications of this shitty disease and more interested in identifying the molecular mechanisms that allow it to form and progress so we can stop it. That's the goal, and I'm pretty sure even philosophers would agree that this goal is the ultimate goal, especially if said philosophers had tumors growing in their boobs.

To understand the how, we need a basic framework for understanding cellular function and its regulation at the molecular level. Don't get bogged down in the terms: *Cellular function* refers to how the cell does its specific job, how it grows and divides, and how it dies—the same basic life cycle that the human host experiences. *Regulation at the molecular level* refers to the plan the cell follows—the blueprint for its growth, function, and death. It starts with *DNA* (deoxyribonucleic acid) molecules, the genetic blueprint in all cells that contains the instructions for the cell's functions and life plan.

So, what does DNA actually do? Or perhaps the better question is, how does the information encoded in DNA molecules actually tell cells what to do? This gets into something called *the central dogma of molecular biology.* That's a fancy-schmancy title for the way in which the instructions encoded in DNA are used to manufacture proteins, the workhorses of cells. When most people think about proteins, they envision a juicy piece of meat or powerful muscles; and the components used to build muscle fibers are, in fact, proteins. But proteins are much more than that: they are the essential building blocks of cells, which in turn build tissues, organs, and all parts of the body. Proteins can be structural, like the fibers that form the cell's cytoskeleton and the histone proteins that wrap around DNA strands and protect them. They can be functional, forming enzymes that do important jobs like metabolizing nutrients, breaking them down into usable building blocks for building biomass and generating energy for the cell. They also play a critical role in transmitting information within cells and between cells, integrating communication between different parts of the body.

Proteins are made up of chains of amino acids, and the order in which they are put together is determined by the sequence of nucleotides in the portion of DNA that encodes that protein. That sequence is called a *gene*. The nucleotides are the chemical components of DNA and include adenine, cytosine, thymine, and guanine—which are abbreviated as A, C, T, and G. A unit of genetic code—called a *codon*—consists of three nucleotides. A sequence of codons contains the information a cell uses to make each protein. But as a matter of practicality, since DNA is housed in a subcellular organelle called the nucleus and is therefore inaccessible to the protein-production machinery in the cytoplasm, and because the cell needs to protect the integrity of its DNA, proteins are not built using pieces of actual DNA. The portion of the DNA, the gene, that encodes instructions for making a specific protein is first transcribed into an intermediate molecule, call *messenger ribonucleic acid* (or *mRNA*; see figure 2.1). Transcriptional machinery within the nucleus unwinds and separates the DNA strands, using one strand to copy the information necessary to build a protein. The mRNA molecule is then transported out of the nucleus (also illustrated in figure 2.1) where it is used by the protein-synthesis machinery to translate the information encoded by the mRNA into protein (as illustrated in figure 2.1). Each amino acid has its own three-nucleotide code, and the protein-synthesis machinery puts amino acids in the order dictated by the code within mRNA molecules. That's the central dogma of molecular biology: DNA is transcribed to RNA, and RNA is translated to protein. The shorthand version of this concept is *DNA to RNA to protein*. After additional folding and processing by other cellular organelles, the mature protein is transported within the

Protein synthesis

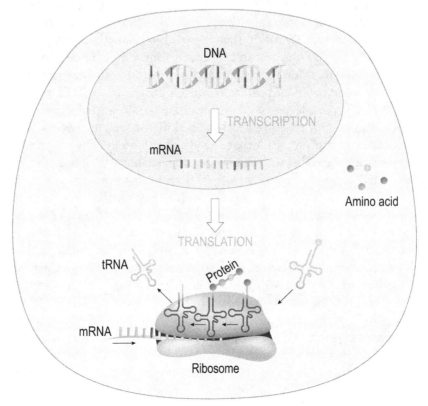

Figure 2.1. Protein synthesis, the central dogma of molecular biology. *Source:* © iStock / ttsz.

cell (and in some cases exported out of the cell) to perform its function. Functions include creating the scaffolding that maintains a cell's structure, becoming enzymes that perform chemical reactions necessary for a cell to stay alive, making copies of itself and dividing, and performing specific tasks required by the tissue and organ of which it is a part to keep the entire body working.[6]

What does all this have to do with cancer? Turns out, quite a lot. Since proteins do pretty much everything a cell needs to function, from actually performing the function to providing the cellular infrastructure and building the cellular machinery that keeps the cell running, it stands to reason that proteins drive cancer. And that's exactly what happens.

But how?

If cancer is your body betraying you in the form of an abnormal growth, then it's controlled by abnormal proteins that were once normal proteins. Most of the proteins that drive cancer are proteins that regulate *cellular division* and *cellular survival*, and they fall into two basic categories: *oncoproteins* and *tumor suppressors*. Oncoproteins are hyperactive. No, scratch that—they're like rabid monkeys on cocaine in terms of uncontrolled activity. These proteins start out as normal proteins, encoded by normal genes—proto-oncogenes. They become oncogenes due to changes in DNA, including (1) point mutations, or changes in nucleotide sequence that change the amino acid encoded and subsequently the activity of the protein, (2) amplification of genes, such that multiple copies make higher than normal levels of the protein, and (3) translocations, which move pieces of DNA around, stitch them together, and make Frankenproteins that wreak havoc on normal cellular function, particularly the molecular pathways that control cell division and susceptibility to programmed cell death. Tumor suppressors, on the other hand, become silenced through DNA alterations, including mutations, deletions, and changes to the accessibility of the tumor-suppressor gene to transcriptional machinery; if the gene cannot be transcribed, there's no messenger RNA to translate and, as a consequence, no protein.

Alterations in DNA-encoding proto-oncogenes and tumor suppressors are major mechanisms that contribute to *malignant transformation*—or the change from a normal cell into a cancer cell. So, it's no surprise that defects in the cellular machinery regulating DNA replication (copy making) and repair (proofreading and correction) contribute to DNA alterations in several types of cancer. DNA can also be damaged by *carcinogens*—or substances that promote the formation of cancer. Some well-known carcinogens include components of cigarette smoke, ultraviolet light from the sun, radiation, and asbestos, all of which can cause DNA damage that, if it occurs in an oncogene and/or a tumor suppressor, can contribute to cancer.

Whether these mutations are caused by random mistakes that occur when DNA is replicated (or copied) before a cell divides (makes a copy of itself) or they're caused by external factors like carcinogens, if these mutations or other alterations are not repaired, and if they occur in a proto-oncogene or tumor suppressor, then they can contribute to cancer. (The video referenced earlier, in note 6, also offers a great explanation.) There are some hereditary or familial cancers that are caused by gene variants being passed from generation to generation—like breast cancer (BRCA) genes 1 and 2[7]—but most breast cancers and most cancers in general are caused by random mutation in cells (tumor-genomic changes that produce sporadic cancers) rather than by heredity (that is, rather than by genetic variants inherited from your parents that predispose you to cancer or increase your cancer risk).

Combinations of mutations and genetic alterations in a once-normal cell can lead to malignant transformation.[8] It usually takes more than one alteration, or "hit," in proto-oncogenes and tumor-suppressor genes to change a cell from a normal but overgrowing cell into cancer. For breast cancer, the number of mutations required to transform a normal breast epithelial cell is four. Since there are so many potential oncogenes and tumor suppressors, not to mention other genes that drive cancer (e.g., genes that control movement, the ability to recruit blood vessels, and interactions with host cells, including immune cells), it makes sense that what causes and promotes cancer in cells is really extra super complex:

1. There are many gene products that work in interconnected *molecular pathways* that regulate cell division and growth, cell movement, and cell communication with other cells and host tissues.
2. Like any well-designed, elegant machine, cells have backup systems should one or more of these pathways fail.
3. Most cancers aren't driven by a single altered genetic/molecular signaling pathway. Most harbor mutations and alterations in many oncogenes, tumor suppressors, and other relevant "driver" molecules, and there are many combinations that make cancer, well, *cancer.*

In a nutshell, cancer isn't a single disease.

Breaking that down even further, breast cancer is not a single disease. It is a collection of diseases that are complex at the molecular-genetic level, adaptable due to genetic instability, and thus extremely difficult to treat and prone to becoming resistant (e.g., nonresponsive to drugs used to keep it at bay; I'll talk more about molecularly targeted therapies and drug resistance later). We will never cure "the cancer" because "the cancer" doesn't exist. It's actually "the cancers," and they are insidious.[9] That being said, there are patterns behind genetic changes and other alterations that make normal cells turn into cancer cells, and these patterns have allowed scientists and clinicians to classify different subtypes of breast cancer based on histopathologic (how breast tumors look under a microscope) and molecular-genetic features (alterations in common driver genes), as discussed below.

Breast Cancer Subtypes

Even before sequencing of the human genome and the revolution of molecular genetics, scientists and clinicians recognized that not all breast cancers look the same under a microscope. Pathologists—medical doctors specializing in the research and testing of medical specimens for the diagnosis and treatment of disease—are meticulous human beings who have been trained to recognize details. They noticed differences between breast-tumor tissue taken from individual patients and categorized them using old-school (but still very much relevant and still used today) *histologic* criteria—how a thin slice through the tumor looks under a microscope. These criteria include size (how big the tumor is), shape (whether or not the tumor is confined by clear boundaries or has invaded into the surrounding healthy tissue), and grade (how fast the tumor cells are dividing, and thus how fast the tumor is growing). Within this classification system, there are at least four types of breast cancer, named for the disease stage and the type of breast cancer:

- Ductal carcinoma in situ, or DCIS
- Invasive ductal carcinoma, or IDC

- Inflammatory breast cancer, or IBC
- Metastatic breast cancer, or MBC.[10]

Breast cancers that originate in the lobular breast epithelium of the breast, the future milk-producing cells at the ends of ducts, can be classified as

- Lobular carcinoma in situ, or LCIS
- Invasive lobular carcinoma, or ILC.[11]

See table 2.1 for more information about the histologic classification system.

With the advent of modern molecular genetics, scientists and pathologists have been able to look at and compare tumor-genomic profiles (meaning they've been able to sequence DNA isolated from tumors and look for changes in normal genes). Some of these genomic profiles include mutations and alterations in tumor DNA that benefit the cancer, and others include levels of gene expression (mRNA and protein) for gene products that benefit the cancer. By analyzing tumor samples from thousands of breast cancer patients, patterns have emerged that helped identify and categorize individual breast cancers with similar characteristics. This led to a new classification system called the *molecular subtype*.

Currently there are four to five distinct molecular subtypes of breast cancer cells, including

- Hormone-receptor-positive/HER2-negative (HR+/HER2–). *Hormone receptor* refers to the estrogen receptor (ER) and progesterone receptor (PR), and *HER2* refers to the HER2 oncogene (all of which will be discussed in greater detail in chapter 4). This type is also known as *Luminal A breast cancer*.
- HR–/HER2–, also known as *triple-negative breast cancer* (TNBC)
- HR+/HER2+, also known as *Luminal B breast cancer*
- and HR–/HER2+, also known as *HER2-enriched breast cancer*.[12]

The fifth subtype, which accounts for approximately 10 percent of all breast cancer cases, is classified as *unknown*, meaning molecular altera-

Table 2.1. Breast cancer stages and their characteristics.

Breast cancer type	Stage	Size of primary tumor	Local invasion?	Distant metastasis?
Ductal carcinoma in situ (DCIS) and lobular carcinoma in situ (LCIS)*	0	>2 cm	No	No
Invasive ductal carcinoma (IDC)	I to III	≥2 cm (stage I)	No (stage IA)	No
		2 to 5 cm stage II)	Yes (stage IB to II)— Regional lymph nodes	No
Invasive lobular carcinoma (ILC)*		2 to >5 cm (stage III)	Yes (stage III)— Regional lymph nodes + lymph nodes near breast bone and/or above collar bone	No
Inflammatory breast cancer (IBC)	III	2 to >5 cm	Yes—Spread to skin of breast	No
Metastatic breast cancer (MBC)	IV	n/a	Yes—Spread beyond breast and regional lymph nodes	Yes—Spread to distant organs (e.g., liver, lung, bone, brain)

* Lobular breast cancers originate in lobular mammary epithelial cells, the precursors of milk-producing cells at the ends of the ductal glandular network.

tions in these breast cancers don't fit neatly into any of the other breast cancer categories. A combination of these two classification systems is used to diagnose individual breast cancers and to make treatment decisions.

Okay, now, hold on to your hats, because it gets even more complicated.

There are subtypes within those molecular subtypes. Or is it sub-sub-types? Hell, I don't even know, and I work in the field. I get a headache sometimes trying to wrap my brain around these Russian nesting-doll levels of complexity. But, trust me, it's great information to have. So, for the HR−/HER2−, aka triple-negative breast cancer subtype, deeper molecular-genetic and gene-expression analyses have revealed patterns that allowed scientists and clinicians to further categorize this subtype of breast cancer into sub(sub)types:

- Basal-like 1 (BL1)
- Basal-like 2 (BL2)
- Mesenchymal and mesenchymal stem–like (M, MSL)
- Luminal-androgen receptor (LAR)
- Immune modulatory (IM). The IM subtype is divided into IM-negative (IM−) or IM-positive (IM+).[13]

What does all of this subtyping mean? For starters, it has allowed scientists and clinicians to predict which patients are at greater risk of poor clinical outcomes based on their subtype. For example, patients with BL1 TNBC tend to respond better to standard chemotherapy (one of the only treatments we currently have for this breast cancer subtype; see chapter 5) than do those with BL2 TNBC, so BL2 patients probably shouldn't get chemotherapy if the risks and side effects outweigh the benefits. BL1 and M subtypes tend to track with mutations in BRCA1, which means they may respond to drugs that target a regulator of DNA damage repair and lead to tumor cell death (e.g., PARP inhibitors; see chapter 5). The IM subtype and the IM-positive sub(sub-sub)type in particular may benefit from new drugs that harness the power of the patient's own immune system to combat the disease (e.g., immune-checkpoint inhibitors; see chapter 16).

In summary, having this detailed information about the stage, grade, and histologic and molecular subtypes for individual breast cancer cases gives clinicians crucial information for making treatment decisions. Knowing what drives each individual breast cancer gives health-care providers more options for treatment, both FDA-approved treatments and treatments being tested in clinical trials. For certain types of breast cancer, this subtyping has also made it possible for a health-care team to predict how likely their patient is to benefit from chemotherapy and to predict the patient's risk of recurrence (i.e., the cancer coming back). (More on those diagnostic tools in chapter 3.)

Metastasis: The Last Stage of Cancer

The molecular and genetic processes that cause mutations, amplifications, deletions, and other abnormalities in DNA continue as long as breast cancer cells live, survive, and divide. Each division represents a new opportunity for DNA changes, some of which help the new daughter cells become more malignant. For cancer cells exposed to treatments like chemotherapy, radiation, and molecularly targeted therapies, or for tumor cells buried deep within the tumor mass in a region with little oxygen or nutrients, small populations of cells that survive become stronger through an artificial evolutionary process. When we think of evolution, we think of Darwin's theory of evolution by *natural selection*—in which traits that give living things an advantage in their environment are more likely to be passed down to future generations. For example, cells with mutations allowing them to divide without being told are more likely to reproduce and pass these mutations, which gives these cells an advantage, to daughter cells. Instead of serving as a pressure for natural selection, therapy puts artificial selective pressure on cells. Those cells with mutations allowing them to survive chemotherapy, radiation, or molecularly targeted therapies can pass those advantageous mutations on to their daughter cells, which then become therapy-resistant.[14]

Over time, additional mutations arise that provide new advantages to the cancer cells. Cells that survive long enough develop changes that allow them to invade, which means they break away from the primary tumor mass and start moving into the surrounding healthy tissue, looking for new places to grow. These cells can enter blood vessels or lymphatic vessels, which puts them into circulation where they can travel throughout the host's body, exit circulation into a new organ, and set up shop and form secondary tumors called *metastases*. Cancer cells have to overcome a *lot* of challenges to get to this stage. Surviving in circulation means withstanding varying fluid pressures in large and small blood vessels, surviving a harsh, foreign environment that breast epithelial cells were never meant to experience, evading circulating immune cells, and settling in a new, foreign environment.[15]

Enduring what amounts to a decathlon, the cells that colonize other organs and form secondary tumors, or metastases, are tough. By this stage, they are often unresponsive to chemotherapy, radiation, or molecularly targeted therapies. If they do respond, metastatic tumors often quickly become resistant due to their genetic instability and the selective pressure. By growing and stealing nutrients from the organ host, metastatic tumors cause organ failure. Lung metastases interfere with breathing and make it difficult to recover from pneumonia. Liver metastases can no longer filter toxins from the body. Metastases in the bone, in addition to weakening bones and increasing the risk for fractures and breaks, can cause excess calcium to be released into the bloodstream. This interferes with heart, kidney, and muscle function, and elevated calcium levels can cause coma or death. Destruction of bone marrow by metastatic tumors also interferes with production of blood cells and immune cells. In the brain, metastatic tumor cells traveling through blood vessels can cause stroke. The holy grail of cancer research is to predict, prevent, and/or successfully treat metastatic breast cancer.

The Beginning of My Career in Breast Cancer Research

I entered the breast cancer research field in 1995 as a graduate student, during the heyday of the molecular-genetic revolution. In the field of breast cancer, the BRCA genes had recently been identified and cloned, meaning that the DNA sequences encoding these genes had been pulled out of their native human DNA context and placed in DNA vectors for rapid, large-scale production that allows scientists to study their functions in a laboratory setting. These BRCA genes encode DNA repair proteins, the loss of which enables mutations in DNA that drive breast and ovarian cancers. These are also genes associated with *familial cancers*—cancers for which a genetic predisposition to breast and ovarian cancer are inherited.

This brings up an important distinction: genetics versus genomics and hereditary cancers versus spontaneous cancers. *Hereditary cancers*, which are relatively rare, run in families due to a genetic defect inherited from one or both parents that exists in every cell in the body. This leaves the person carrying the mutation with a genetic predisposition to developing cancer, like women who carry mutant BRCA genes. By contrast, *spontaneous cancers*, which make up most cancer cases, including breast cancer cases, are caused by mutations that occur in future cancer cells in one part of the body rather than a mutation that exists in every cell; these mutations are acquired later in life rather than being present at conception.

I got to witness many exciting developments in the field during my training. The Human Genome Project was in progress. Development of *microarray profiling*—a revolutionary technique that allows quantification and comparison of gene expression at the level of messenger RNA—enabled molecular classification of tumors. This research was the basis for classifying breast cancers into distinct molecular subtypes. This work also led to publicly available, searchable datasets that allow researchers to compare findings in their laboratory cell- and animal-model systems to data from human cancers in order to establish clinical relevance. Herceptin, the first molecularly targeted therapy developed for HER2+ breast cancers, was saving women who had this aggressive breast cancer subtype, and the FDA had approved the first aromatase inhibitor for use in postmenopausal women with estrogen-receptor-positive disease. This class of drugs, which block estrogen production in the body, has become a standard of care for ER+ disease. (I'll cover these drugs more in chapter 5.) RNA-interference technology—in which gene expression is knocked down by using artificial small interfering RNA molecules to highjack the cellular machinery that uses microRNA to attenuate gene expression—allowed unprecedented molecular-genetic studies in cell lines and in whole-animal models.

It was an exciting time to be a scientist.

Good thing, since this excitement is what got me through the five grueling, wonderful, terrible, disheartening, hopeful, and really fucking challenging years I spent as a graduate student. I didn't come from a long line of scholars. I wasn't the first in my family to go to college, but I was the first to finish. I was a former high school slacker with a bad attitude who did a one-eighty and made good in college when I got my ass in gear and brought my A game. That theme continued into graduate school. I was the first in my family to pursue a postgraduate degree, and I understood on a visceral level how damned lucky I was to have the opportunity to train at a world-class academic-research institution.

That understanding made me a hard-working, nose-to-the-grindstone, relentlessly dedicated student.

It also chiseled a really huge chip on my shoulder, due to a dangerous combination of untreated anxiety, imposter syndrome, and a whole lot of rage that did not serve me well in my early twenties. I was not alone; women in academics have always faced an uphill battle—kind of like women in general. As I mentioned in the introduction to this book, the patriarchy is very real, and it is, sadly, still thriving in academics (more on that in chapter 12). Yes, things are getting better—if you're a cis, heterosexual White woman. But we still have a lot of work to do to create access and parity among all groups of people, regardless of skin color and gender. These challenges are mirrored in the challenges breast cancer patients face when seeking health care and support: Most breast cancer patients are female—though men can be diagnosed as well—so sexism and the patriarchy are two hurdles patients must clear. If you're poor, add another hurdle. If you're not White, add about five hurdles (more on this in chapter 6). If you're not straight, add a couple of hurdles. If you're disabled, add in three flights of stairs and no ramp. If you're trans, throw in a fifty-foot wall between you and access to fair, equitable health care.

I'll talk more about sexism in academics and the health-care system later, and I have a whole lot to say about disparities in health care for marginalized groups. But first, since we're here to talk about breast cancer, the next chapter covers what to do if you're one of the one in eight women diagnosed with breast cancer. This important discussion is also relevant for any human being diagnosed with breast cancer. Knowledge is power, and it can save your life.

CHAPTER THREE

~

Diagnostics

Imaging, Poking, and Prodding to Find Breast Cancer

"You have cancer."

Those are three words no one ever wants to hear. But the fact is that for 284,200 people this year alone, these words are inescapable.[1] And they are terrifying. I'll detail my personal story and reaction to a breast cancer diagnosis in chapter 7, but first I want to dive deep into the nuts and bolts of *diagnostic tools*, including mammography, breast MRI imaging, breast ultrasounds, and biopsies aided by mammography, ultrasound, and MRI. Using stage, grade, and subtype information discussed in chapter 2, chapter 4 will cover *treatment decisions* that include surgery, chemotherapy, and/or radiation therapy, as well as molecularly targeted therapies. Chapter 4 will also cover Oncotype DX and MammaPrint *gene-expression-profiling tests*, as well as specialized testing by Foundation Medicine, and there we'll discuss how these diagnostic and prognostic tools have revolutionized treatment options for certain subtypes of breast cancer.

If you're a patient who's ever heard the words *you have cancer*, I want you to take a moment and breathe. Take a deep breath in through your nose, hold it for four seconds, and then slowly exhale for about four seconds through your nose or mouth. Repeat this until your heart rate slows, the tightness in your chest loosens, your hands stop shaking, and you can think again. Do this each time panic threatens to drown you in a sea of fear and uncertainty.

Better? Good.

First thing to know—and this is super important—you are not alone. You are now part of an exclusive club that none of us wanted to join but binds us together in solidarity and support. The survivor community is full of incredible people who've been through or are going through what you are about to experience. They are an invaluable resource, and they are generous in their advice and support. I've provided links to places where you can connect with survivors, and I encourage you to ask your medical-care team about resources in your community.

Your health-care team will order a battery of diagnostic tests to determine your breast cancer stage, grade, and histologic/molecular subtype and to identify the mutations that are driving your cancer. These tools will help them, and you, determine how best to treat it. So, let's get started with the *diagnostic tools* that your health-care team might order for you.

Diagnostic Tools

If you've received a breast cancer diagnosis, odds are you've had mammograms, MRI imaging, ultrasound imaging, and some type of biopsy. I've had them all. If you haven't experienced any or all of these yet, let me break down each of these procedures so you'll know what to expect. I'll spill the tea about my personal experiences in greater detail in chapters 7 and 8. Bear in mind that each medical center and care team has its own protocols, and your experience may differ, but this overview should give you an idea about the purpose of each diagnostic test and what you'll see, hear, feel, and maybe smell.

Yes, *smell*.

I swear I can smell the ultrasound jelly, and even though it's supposed to smell like alcohol, since that's its primary ingredient, it smells like spray-on sunscreen to me.

Okay, let's start with the *mammogram*. It's a specialized type of X-ray that allows the inside of breast tissue to be seen by *radiologists*—the medical doctors who specialize in diagnosing and treating injuries and diseases using medical imaging. X-rays are a form of radiation—

electromagnetic waves that are absorbed or passed through different parts of your body, which creates an internal image that can be used for diagnostics. You can see mine in figure 3.1. The images produced highlight areas of high tissue density, masses, and calcifications that may be signs of cancer.[2]

When should a person start getting mammograms, and are mammograms really necessary? It turns out, the answers to these questions depend on which agency you believe. Guidelines curated by the Centers for Disease Control recommend screenings for women beginning

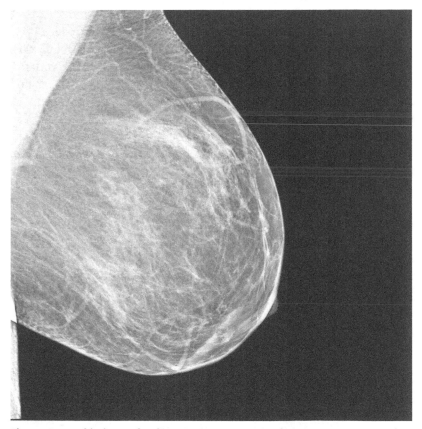

Figure 3.1. This is my boob on a mammogram. *Source:* **Dana M. Brantley-Sieders, mammogram part of my medical record.**

between the ages forty and fifty, anywhere from once a year to once every two years through age seventy-five or to the end of the patient's life.[3] Women who have risk factors such as a family history of breast cancer, mutations in the BRCA1 or BRCA2 genes, and/or a history of mantle radiation (an older method for treating Hodgkin lymphoma) or chest radiation that occurred before age thirty should talk to their health-care providers about the frequency of mammography screening.

So, what should you do? My best advice is to speak with your health-care provider about the risks and benefits of mammography and your personal risk of breast cancer so that you can decide what's best for you. That being said, my stage Ib IDC (invasive ductal carcinoma) breast cancer was detected by routine mammogram when I was forty-five. Had I waited until I was fifty to get screened, I'd likely have been diagnosed with stage III or IV breast cancer after finding a palpable lump, or I might even be dead now. I do not have any common genetic variants associated with breast cancer or any other type of cancer. I personally am a proponent of screening starting at age forty, but, again, in order to make the best decision for you, talk to your health-care team, and maybe even seek out advice from other providers. Make sure you provide as much information about any breast or ovarian cancers that have been diagnosed in your DNA relatives, and ask your care team about other factors that might put you at a higher risk for breast cancer, including age, reproductive history (including the age at which you got your first period and, if applicable, the age at which you entered menopause), breast-tissue density, genetic mutations like BRCA1 and -2, exposure to hormones (e.g., hormone-replacement therapy, or HRT), other breast issues (e.g., noncancerous breast diseases), previous exposure to radiation and certain drugs, physical activity, weight and BMI, alcohol use, and other lifestyle factors.[4] Bear in mind that mammography can miss up to 20 percent of breast cancers that are present at the time of screening. This can be due to high breast density, and false negatives occur more often in younger women. In addition to false negatives, unfortunately some breast cancers grow so rapidly that they can appear within months of a normal mammogram. Remember to keep up with breast self-exams.[5] Contact your health-care providers with any concerns, and bear in mind that some cancers not detected by mammograms can be detected by clinical breast exams—like the ones you normally get at your annual checkup with your gynecologist.[6]

Here's what to expect from a mammography exam: You'll be led from the waiting room of your provider's office to a waiting area that may or may not have other patients waiting for their mammograms. You'll be given a robe or smock and asked to remove your clothing from the waist up, and you'll put on the robe or smock to "preserve modesty." This is so your tits won't be on display—like that time my husband convinced me to drop 'em out on a beach in Europe (he's European). Like, hello, Babe, I'm American and I was raised Southern Baptist, we don't *do* that sort of thing . . . unless, oh, I don't know, our husband wheedles, needles, and cajoles us until we yell, "Fine, here ya go!" and then proceed to pull down the top of our one-piece suit (which was also a source of humor for hubby and most other scantily clad bikini- and banana hammock–wearing folks on the beach) on a desolate road on the way back to the hotel.

Anyway, I digress.

At your mammogram appointment, you'll sit in one of the waiting room chairs and wait to be called. When it's your turn, the mammography technician will call you in, hopefully introduce themselves and smile to put you at ease, and then go over what they'll be doing during the procedure. You'll most likely get a digital mammography scan, possibly 3D mammography, one boob at a time. You aren't supposed to wear deodorant to the exam (the aluminum particles in deodorant can mess up the reading, since they can look like calcifications in the image). I always forget, so I have to use the wipes provided by the office to clean off my pits. If your exam is scheduled for a hot, muggy summer day, you might want to bring deodorant with you so you can reapply when you're done.

The technician will help situate you by placing your breast between two plastic trays and clamping down on what is basically a vise to squeeze and hold your breast in place. This isn't just some sick torture thing; X-rays don't pass easily through breast tissue, so compression helps spread the tissue apart to create a clear image. Working as quickly as they can, they will move to the computer, ask you to hold your breath (this will keep your breast from moving, helping to get a clear image) for around five to ten seconds, and then they'll tell you to breathe and will release your breast from compression. You'll repeat this process a few times so the technician can get images of your breast from different angles. If your mammography is a routine exam, you'll get both breasts done. If the exam is a follow-up, you may only get images taken from the breast with the suspicious spot. In general, the exam takes about fifteen to thirty minutes.

After the technician is satisfied with the number and quality of images, you'll either be asked to stay in the mammography room while the images are shown to the radiologist, or the tech will ask you to wait back in the common waiting area with other smocked/robed women. If you're like me, a woman who has been called back because they found something every freaking time since you started getting mammograms, you'll probably be a bit nervous or panicky. I recommend deep breathing exercises, funny cat videos on YouTube, surfing Facebook/Twitter/Instagram/Snapchat/TikTok/whatever else is out there shortly after this book is published, or using your time to update your Pinterest boards. You can also bring a juicy, smutty romance novel or browse a magazine. I also recommend having a text buddy to help take your mind off the agony of waiting. This is where living in the digital age comes in handy; I'm not sure I would have done as well without e-distractions.

Hopefully the technician will come back in and tell you you're all clear and that they'll see you next year. If they don't, don't panic; most of the time, it's nothing. The first three callbacks I got after suspicious mammograms ended up being nothing to be super concerned about. Something that's baseline suspicious and merits a follow-up scan could turn out to be nothing more than a cyst, a fibroadenoma, fat necrosis, an area of breast density that merits surveillance but not immediate attention, or simply an ambiguous or bad image that can be resolved with a do-over.

And if it *does* turn out to be something important that's shown up on the imaging, it's better to tackle it sooner rather than later. Believe me.

Mammograms aren't fun. Putting your boob in a glorified vise that flattens it may help get better images, but it sure as hell isn't comfortable. When they get closer to the chest wall, it's even more uncomfortable. The technicians and radiologists should be and are—at least in my experience—kind and will do everything they can to make the process as quick as possible and minimize discomfort. Taking painkillers prior to a mammogram helps. Joking with your mammography technician and radiologist helps too—at least for me.

If the mammography technician and radiologist see something suspicious on a mammogram, they'll usually take more mammography images as a first step in order to get a better look. They may also order an *MRI scan*. Magnetic resonance imaging uses a magnetic field and computer-generated radio waves to produce high-resolution images of organs and tissues deep within the body. The magnetic field makes protons (*High school science review:* protons are positively charged subatomic particles present in atoms, which make up everything including your body) of hydrogen atoms align with the magnetic field. The beam of radio waves stimulates the protons to strain against the pull of the magnetic field, and the data from this tug of war is used to create digital images. It's very cool. While I don't have any of my own MRI images, figure 3.2 is a photograph of a breast MRI to show you what your health-care team sees.

In terms of preparation for a breast MRI, you are generally asked to lay on your stomach on a cushioned table attached to the MRI machine, and your breasts are fitted into holes in the table, leaving them to hang below. These holes—or depressions—contain detectors for the magnetic signals. You'll likely be given a contrast agent (a dye—e.g., gadolinium) through an IV to make the images clearer and easier to

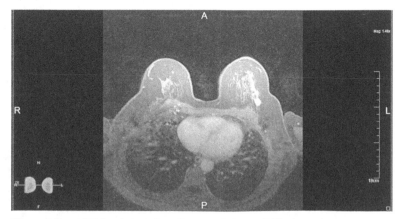

Figure 3.2.   MRI boob imaging. *Source:* © **Deposit Photos.**

interpret. Make sure your health-care team and the MRI technicians know about any allergies you have and if you have kidney issues, since the dye can cause an allergic reaction or cause problems with already-compromised kidney function.

Some other things to consider before getting an MRI:

- Schedule your MRI at the beginning of your menstrual cycle, if you have them (e.g., between days three and fourteen, where day one is the first day you bleed on your period).
- Make sure you have no metal on your body at the time of the scan, since it could react with the magnet, and tell your health-care team about any metal devices inside your body (e.g., pacemaker, defibrillator, implanted drug port, or artificial joint).
- If you're pregnant, the gadolinium contrast dye could pose a risk to the baby, so MRI isn't generally recommended.
- Even though the dye poses very little risk, if you're nursing you may want to bank breast milk before your MRI and stop breastfeeding for two days after your MRI to make sure the contrast dye is gone.

In order for the tech to generate the magnetic field in a controlled way, you'll be wheeled into a tube. If you're claustrophobic, talk to your health-care team and the MRI technician. It is important that you breathe normally and lie as still as possible during the imaging process, and you may be able to get a mild sedative to make the process less stressful. You'll also be given earplugs, since the machine is freaking loud, with lots of thumps and taps, but you'll still be able to hear and speak to the MRI technician throughout the exam. The imaging takes anywhere from thirty minutes to an hour. I'm weird (as you've probably guessed by now), so I actually fell asleep during my MRI exam; after years of graduate school, postdoctoral training, babies that grew into kids, and the march into middle age, I've learned to nap when and where I can (don't judge). Once you're done, you'll get dressed and go about your daily routine until your health-care team contacts you about the results.

The waiting is the hardest part.

Your health-care team will review the images and determine if additional images and/or a biopsy are warranted (see below for biopsies).

MRIs are not a substitute for mammograms. Mammograms are first on the list of diagnostic-imaging tools for breast, followed by breast MRI and breast ultrasounds (which I cover below). MRI imaging comes with the risk of false positives, meaning that a suspicious spot identified on the MRI may result in breast ultrasound and biopsy that ultimately determines that the spot is benign; as I've learned from personal experience, that's pretty stressful. The other risk for MRI is a potential reaction to the contrast dye. In spite of these risks, MRI imaging can complement mammography and give your health-care team more information to determine the best course of action when they identify an abnormality in your breast.[7]

Your health-care team may also order an *ultrasound*. Most of us are familiar with ultrasound in the context of pregnancy, since this imaging method is routinely used to check on the health and development of a fetus at least once during pregnancy. Ultrasound is a form of *sonography*, an imaging method using sound waves that penetrate soft tissue and liquid and then bounce off denser tissue. The sound-wave echoes can be detected and translated into an image of the internal structures of the area being probed. In the case of a breast ultrasound, the sound waves travel through the skin and into the fatty tissue, creating echoes that are converted into electrical signals by a detector, which a computer then uses to construct points of brightness on the image. You can see mine in figure 3.3, which shows a side-by-side comparison of a benign lesion detected in my right breast (left) prior to imaging that helped detect the tumor in my left breast (right).

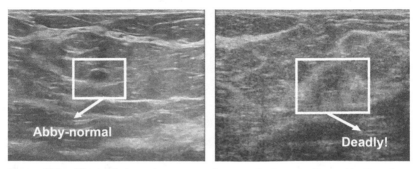

Figure 3.3.   The weird spots on my ultrasound. *Source:* Dana M. Brantley-Sieders, ultrasounds part of my medical record.

Preparation for an ultrasound is much the same as preparation for a mammogram: The technician will ask you to recline on a hospital bed or gurney and have you expose the boob they want to image. You can keep the other one covered with your robe, and the tech will cover you with a cloth when they leave to consult with the radiologist. The technician will apply ultrasound jelly to the ultrasound wand (the wide stick thingy they'll press against your breast) and may also apply some to your breast. If you're lucky, the jelly will be warmed up; otherwise, it'll be a wee bit chilly. Depending on the region the technician needs to scan, they may ask you to hold your hand over your head so they can access more of the breast tissue. You can rest it on a pillow. When it starts to go numb or get sore, let the tech know, and they'll happily let you take a break—or, at least, they should. Don't be afraid to speak up. These techs are some of the most compassionate people on the planet, and they do not want you to be uncomfortable.

The technician will place the wand on your breast and slide it around to look for the area of interest. They'll press down sometimes to view deeper tissue, and then they'll slowly release pressure, repeating the process several times when they've found the correct spot. This shouldn't hurt. After finding the correct spot, the tech will take digital photographs, and then they'll give you a cloth to remove the jelly from your skin and cover you while they consult with the radiologist. The exam usually takes fifteen to thirty minutes.[8]

The lights are generally low in ultrasound suites, and I've actually fallen asleep twice while waiting for the technician to return, much as I did during my MRI exams. (Yeah, I'm a weirdo. I'm also a working mom. I sleep whenever and wherever I can.)

The radiologist will often enter the room, review the images captured by the ultrasound technician, and possibly repeat the exam to get a better look. The radiologist will then discuss the results with you. They may suggest a follow-up scan to monitor the suspicious spot, or they may recommend a *biopsy*. This involves taking a small tissue sample from the area of interest for analysis by a pathologist (remember, that's the physician who specializes in examining body fluids and tissues to diagnose medical problems). Using imaging methods described above, the radiologist will find the area of interest and insert a needle to extract portions of tissue in the area for analysis by a pathologist.

Don't freak out. Before inserting the needle, the radiologist admin-isters local anesthetic to make sure your breast is numb. During my ultrasound- and mammogram-guided biopsies, I experienced pressure but no pain. For me the biggest discomfort for the mammogram-guided biopsy was having to lie facedown on a table and stay still for about fifteen minutes. I'm a wiggler; it was tough. Also, I'm pushing fifty, so prone positions without cushioning tend to amplify all of my age-related aches and pains. Again, I recommend taking painkillers before a biopsy, but be sure and check in with your health-care team first, since some over-the-counter painkillers also function as blood thinners, which could complicate the procedure.

I also appreciated the wonderful nurse who rubbed my back and told me I was doing great throughout the procedure. Kindness and compas-sion go a long way. (Nurses are the best!)

So, the general procedure is as follows: You'll strip from the waist up and go through the motions of getting situated on the gurney (ul-trasound), table or chair (mammogram), or MRI table. The radiologist and technician will image your breast to find the area of interest. Once they've found it, you'll receive a local anesthetic (e.g., lidocaine injec-tion). The radiologist will then use a thin needle to take tissue samples from the area, collecting them into a tube or tubes with preservative, and send them off to a pathologist, who will look for abnormalities to diagnose benign (not cancerous) or malignant (cancerous) disease. The radiologist will then implant a small tissue marker at the biopsy site so the site can be easily located on future mammograms, MRIs, and ultra-sounds, which is especially important for surveillance and to locate the site again if the biopsy reveals cancer. After collecting the samples and inserting the tissue marker, the radiologist will seal the biopsy site with Steri-Strips or surgical glue.

Again, the nurses who were kind enough to reach down and hold my hand during the lidocaine injection and later while the radiologist rooted around in my boob with the needle are the heroes of the health-care sys-tem. I'm a tough cookie, but that small gesture meant the world to me. I also appreciated the radiologists who took the time to squeeze my shoul-der in reassurance after each biopsy. Again, kindness goes a long way.

As with most diagnostic tests, the waiting truly is the hardest part. I've had the crap luck of getting most of my biopsies near the end of the week. Longer wait times equal more stress. Again, distractions help. Once the biopsy results are in, you'll be called into your health-care provider's office to discuss the results. Most of the time you'll find out that the spot is nothing to be concerned about, especially with a Breast Imaging–Reporting and Data System (BI-RADS) score of 3 or lower. BI-RADS is a standardized reporting system for breast imaging that includes mammograms, MRIs, and ultrasounds. Lesion categories 1 through 3 are classified as probably benign, and lesion categories 4 through 6 are suspicious or highly suggestive of cancer. In a 2020 study looking at medical records from over forty-five thousand women with mammography BI-RADS 3 lesions, investigators tracked the number of breast cancers diagnosed after immediate biopsy versus surveillance (i.e., waiting and imaging again after six, twelve, and twenty-four months), and 810 breast cancers were diagnosed—or roughly 2 percent. The majority of breast cancers were diagnosed at or just after the six-month follow-up.[9] *Bottom line:* odds are, the spot is nothing to be concerned about, but if you have a score of 3 or higher, follow up!

Cysts (fluid-filled pockets that can form in the breast), fibroadenomas (benign lesions made up of fibrous tissue), areas of fat necrosis (that can result from traumatic injury, like from seatbelts in a bad car crash), and benign papillomas (painful but noncancerous lesions that can cause nipple discharge) are the most likely culprits for an abnormal scan. If you have dense breast tissue, which tends to be more common in younger women and women with small breasts but can affect any woman, it can be difficult to distinguish problem areas from the fibrous matrix that holds your breasts together.

If you do hear those three dreaded words, *You have cancer,* hold on, breathe, and remember that knowledge is power. In the first two chapters, we covered the basics of how normal breasts function, how normal breast epithelial cells can transform into cancer cells, and how breast cancers are classified based on stage, grade, and molecular profile. The next chapters cover treatment plans—including surgery, chemotherapy, radiation, and molecularly targeted therapies, as well as tumor molecular-profiling tests that have revolutionized how health-care providers work with patients to make the best treatment decisions for each specific breast cancer case.

~

CHAPTER FOUR

Tumor Gene-Expression Profiling and Surgical Options

Excise and Examine

In the previous chapter, we covered diagnostic tools. Once you have a diagnosis of breast cancer, your health-care provider will share details about your tumor's stage, grade, and pathologic and molecular subtype and use that information to recommend treatment options. For some subtypes, tumor gene-expression-profiling tests like Oncotype DX and MammaPrint may be recommended to determine the risk of recurrence (i.e., the cancer coming back) and the likely benefit of chemotherapy. Emerging tools in *personalized medicine*—the concept that treatment decisions should be tailored to each individual patient based on predicted risk and response for disease—are also helpful for making treatment decisions for breast cancer patients, with organizations like Foundation Medicine using advanced methods in tumor genomic- and gene-expression analyses to identify more precise treatment options for patients.

What is tumor gene-expression profiling? It is a technique that involves isolating mRNA from tumor-biopsy tissue or tumor tissue and then analyzing and quantifying the expression levels (e.g., number of mRNA transcripts) for specific genes that are known to make cancer cells grow, survive, and invade. *Remember:* DNA to mRNA to protein. The more mRNA for a cancer-driving Frankenprotein (and less mRNA for tumor-suppressor proteins that put the brakes on growth), the more copies of the protein running amok and wreaking havoc in the form of cancer. These transcript levels are measured against normal "housekeeping-" or reference-mRNA gene products that are common and pretty evenly expressed in all cells, whether the cells are healthy or cancerous. These include mRNAs that gets translated into proteins of the cytoskeleton that gives the cell its shape, glucose and carbohydrate metabolism regulators, iron-uptake regulators, and ribosomal components (part of the protein complex that translates mRNA). These are all essential genes that no cell can live without, including a cancer cell, and their levels don't change in cancer cells. The normalized levels of mRNAs that encode tumor-driver and tumor-suppressor proteins are used to create a recurrence score that is calculated based on clinical research looking for patterns in a large number of tumors from thousands of patients followed for years after their cancer diagnoses and treatments and seeing which genes' expression levels are associated with the cancer coming back (recurrence) with or without chemotherapy. (See below for more details on the Oncotype DX test, the twenty-one gene-panel test most commonly used in the United States. Mamma-Print is a similar seventy-gene panel test used in Europe and also in the United States.)

Tumor-Genomic Testing

Tumor-Genomic testing—which uses gene-expression (see explanation below) profiles in tumors to inform treatment decisions—is one of the most exciting advances in breast cancer clinical oncology. Oncotype DX,[1] which is most commonly used in the United States, is used to predict how likely early-stage estrogen-receptor-positive (ER+) breast cancer is to recur (come back) and whether or not a patient is likely to benefit from chemotherapy after surgery (adjuvant chemotherapy—which means you get the treatment after surgery).

Let's break down what gene-expression profiles (GEPs) are, what tumor-genomic testing can (and cannot) tell us, how they were developed and validated, and their value in the clinic. This is going to be a bit long and involved, but it's important. And I'll do my best to make it comprehensible, informative, and entertaining.

First, let's start with some distinctions between tumor-*genomic* testing and *genetic* testing. *Genetic* testing—such as screening for inherited mutations in BRCA genes that are associated with a *much* higher risk for breast cancer—looks for inherited genetic variants that have been present in the patient's genome since conception and are present in every cell; these variants can be passed on to the patient's children. In other words, you get these genetic variants from your parents. *Genomic* testing looks at patterns of genes that are expressed (i.e., produced) from tumor DNA specifically, which carries acquired mutations that are present in tumor cells but not in other cells in the patient's body and cannot be passed to the patient's children.

Most cancers, including breast cancers, aren't caused by genetically inherited mutations. According to the Centers for Disease Control, only 5 to 10 percent of breast cancers are hereditary.[2]

Background for Gene Expression and Cancer

As we discussed in chapter 2, abnormal gene expression in tumors results from mutations in the genes that regulate cell division and survival. Things that make cancers grow are encoded by oncogenes that often have more copies (amplified in DNA) or make more gene product (increased in mRNA or protein expression). Proteins that stop cancer cells from growing are encoded by tumor-suppressor genes, which get shut down in cancer. Other genes that get mutated or shut down include those that help fix DNA mistakes (DNA repair). DNA damage can lead to more mutations and more copies of bad genes, making cancer worse.

> *Take home:* Genomic testing looks at abnormal gene-expression profiles in *tumors* that are created by (1) amplification or abnormally high expression of oncogenes, which encode positive regulators of cell division and survival, and (2) reduced expression of tumor suppressors, which encode negative regulators of cell division and survival.

The net effect of these mutations, amplifications, and generally messed-up tumor DNA is a radical change in gene expression relative to a normal cell. You might be asking, "What is gene expression, anyway?" Remember the central dogma of molecular biology that we covered in chapter 2? Here's a quick refresher: Genes are encoded in DNA, which is protected in the cell's nucleus and is only unwound during DNA replication (copying) before a cell divides and (in small portions) when genes are *transcribed* into an intermediate, known as mRNA. These copies of mRNA are the templates used by protein-synthesis machinery, which *translates* the genetic code into amino acid chains that eventually form proteins, the workhorses of the cell. This is the central dogma of molecular biology—*DNA to RNA to protein.* We (scientists) use it as the basis of studying how cells behave at the molecular-genetic level.

Development and Validation of Tumor-Genomic Tests

So, tumor-genomic testing assesses gene-expression profiles by measuring mRNA levels—which are higher or lower in cancer cells due to mutation, amplification, or deletion of DNA—and by looking for patterns in a large number of tumors from thousands of patients followed for years after their cancer diagnoses and treatments. Researchers have been able to develop a test based on the gene-expression patterns they discovered when they compared patients who had recurrences (cancers that came back) with patients who didn't have recurrences when they looked at the rates of recurrence for patients who'd had chemotherapy and patients who hadn't. The data were then used to create a *recurrence score* (RS) that can be used to determine (1) the risk of distant recurrence (also referred to as *metastatic recurrence*—or cancer in any part of the body other than where it originated—which is what often kills patients), (2) breast cancer–specific mortality (death from breast cancer) for patients with early-stage ER+ breast cancer, and (3) how likely a patient is to benefit from chemotherapy.

The test is considered more reliable for patients who do not have breast cancer in their lymph nodes,[3] though more recent studies suggest it might be applicable to some lymph node–positive patients.[4] Like many findings in science, however, whether or not this is true depends on whose paper you read and how you interpret the results. Studies are still ongoing to determine whether or not the test can be applied to a broader set of ER+ breast cancers.[5]

Take home: Mutations/amplifications/deletions/alterations in genomic DNA lead to abnormal gene-expression patterns (in
mRNA) that have been identified and used to create a test that
predicts risk of breast cancer coming back, breast cancer death,
and the likely benefit of chemotherapy for early-stage ER+ breast
cancer.

So, what are the gene products measured in the test, and how do
the gene products drive cancer? The panel in the Oncotype DX test
includes twenty-one genes: sixteen tumor genes and five reference
"housekeeping" genes (genes that are not altered in cancers) that were
selected based on decades of laboratory and clinical research. The
genes selected for the panel include

- *Regulators of proliferation.* These are genes that make cells grow.
- *Regulators of invasion.* These are genes that make the cancer move
  out of the primary site and go on to other places in the body.
- *The HER2 group.* The HER2 and associated genes regulate prolif-
  eration and migration—or movement.
- *Estrogen-regulation and -signaling genes.* These are hormones that
  drive breast cancer cell proliferation.
- *Other genes with predictive/prognostic value.*
- And *the reference genes.*

See table 4.1 for a list of genes and more information on what they do.

What the Tumor Gene-Expression-Profiling Tests Can and Cannot Tell Us

Recurrence scores (RS) are based on differential expression of the
genes listed above and are used to classify patients into low-, inter-
mediate-, and high-risk groups; the lower the score, the lower the
risk. The RS provides a *probability* of recurrence based on data from
patients with similar gene-profile patterns. This testing cannot tell you
absolutely whether or not your disease will come back. Similarly, the
test can tell you, based on the outcomes of patients with similar gene
profiles to yours, the probability that you will or will not benefit from
chemotherapy. Given the terrible side effects and long-term effects of
chemotherapy, this information is pretty powerful.

Table 4.1. Genes profiled in the Oncotype DX test and their functions in breast cancer.

Gene	Type of protein encoded	Function in breast cancer
Proliferation regulators[a]		*Make tumor cells divide/tumors grow*
Ki67	DNA-binding protein	Maintains chromosome integrity
STK15	DNA-binding protein	Separates chromosomes
Survivin	DNA-binding protein/inhibitor of cell death	Separates chromosomes; stops cancer cells from dying
Cyclin B1	Kinase-binding protein	Drives cell division forward
MYBL2	Gene-expression regulator	Induces expression of cell-division genes
Invasion regulators[b]		*Make tumor cells spread and metastasize*
Stromelysin 3	Enzyme	Destroys extracellular matrix
Cathepsin L2	Enzyme	Destroys extracellular matrix
HER2 group[c]		Makes tumor cells divide and move/spread
HER2	Signaling receptor	Makes cells grow/move
Grb7	Kinase (HER2)–binding protein	Makes cells grow/move
Estrogen regulators/ signalers[d]		*Make tumor cells divide/tumors grow*
Estrogen receptor (ER)	Gene-expression regulator	Estrogen-induced cell growth
Progesterone receptor (PR)	Gene-expression regulator	Progesterone-induced cell growth
Bcl2	Prosurvival protein	Keeps tumor cells alive
SCUBE2	Proliferation regulator	Stops tumor cell division
Other genes[e]		*Chemotherapy responses, tumor-cell survival*
GSTM1	Enzyme	Detoxifies chemotherapy drugs
BAG1	Prosurvival protein	Keeps tumor cells alive
CD68	Immune-cell marker	Indicates the number of tumor-associated macrophages*
Reference genes		*"Housekeeping" genes not affected by cancer*

Beta Actin	Mostly structural	n/a
GAPDH		
RPLPO		
GUS		
TFRC		

* *Macrophages are a type of immune cell that gets hijacked by tumor cells, leading to suppression of the patient's immune-system response to the cancer tumor, also sometimes being recruited to help the tumor cells invade and metastasize.*

Sources:

a. Xiaoming Sun and Paul D. Kaufman, "Ki-67: More than a Proliferation Marker," *Chromosoma* 127, no. 2 (June 2018): 175–86, https://doi.org/10.1007/s00412-018-0659-8, https://www.ncbi.nlm.nih.gov/pubmed/29322240; Weifeng Tang Hao Qiu et al., "Aurora-A V571 (rs1047972) Polymorphism and Cancer Susceptibility: A Meta-Analysis Involving 27,269 Subjects," *PLoS One* 9, no. 3 (2014): e90328, https://doi.org/10.1371/journal.pone.0090328, https://www.ncbi.nlm.nih.gov/pubmed/24598702; Himani Garg et al., "Survivin: A Unique Target for Tumor Therapy," *Cancer Cell International* 16 (June 23, 2016): 49, https://doi.org/10.1186/s12935-016-0326-1, https://www.ncbi.nlm.nih.gov/pubmed/27340370; Chenyang Ye et al., "Prognostic Role of Cyclin B1 in Solid Tumors: A Meta-Analysis," *Oncotarget* 8, no. 2 (January 10, 2017): 2224–32, https://doi.org/10.18632/oncotarget.13663, https://www.ncbi.nlm.nih.gov/pubmed/27903976; and Julian Musaet al., "MYBL2 (B-Myb): A Central Regulator of Cell Proliferation, Cell Survival and Differentiation Involved in Tumorigenesis," *Cell Death and Disease* 8, no. 6 (June 22, 2017): e2895, https://doi.org/10.1038/cddis.2017.244, https://www.ncbi.nlm.nih.gov/pubmed/28640249.

b. Manoj Kumar Jena and Jagadeesh Janjanam, "Role of Extracellular Matrix in Breast Cancer Development: A Brief Update," *F1000Research* 7 (March 5, 2018): 274, https://doi.org/10.12688/f1000research.14133.2, https://www.ncbi.nlm.nih.gov/pubmed/29983921; and Magdalena Rudzińska et al., "The Role of Cysteine Cathepsins in Cancer Progression and Drug Resistance," *International Journal of Molecular Sciences* 20, no. 14 (July 23, 2019): 3602, https://doi.org/10.3390/ijms20143602, https://www.ncbi.nlm.nih.gov/pubmed/31340550.

c. Jiani Wang and Binghe Xu, "Targeted Therapeutic Options and Future Perspectives for HER2-Positive Breast Cancer," *Signal Transduct and Targeted Therapy* 4 (September 13, 2019): 34, https://doi.org/10.1038/s41392-019-0069-2, https://www.ncbi.nlm.nih.gov/pubmed/31637013; and Yasmine Nadler et al., "Growth Factor Receptor-Bound Protein-7 (Grb7) as a Prognostic Marker and Therapeutic Target in Breast Cancer," *Annals of Oncology* 21, no. 3 (March 2010): 466–73, https://doi.org/10.1093/annonc/mdp346, https://www.ncbi.nlm.nih.gov/pubmed/19717535.

d. Elgee Lim et al., "Pushing Estrogen Receptor Around in Breast Cancer," *Endocrine Related Cancer* 23, no. 12 (December 2016): T227–41, https://doi.org/10.1530/ERC-16-0427, https://www.ncbi.nlm.nih.gov/pubmed/27729416; Cheng-Har Yip and Anthony Rhodes, "Estrogen and Progesterone Receptors in Breast Cancer," *Future Oncology* 10, no. 14 (November 2014): 2293–2301, https://doi.org/10.2217/fon.14.110, https://www.ncbi.nlm.nih.gov/pubmed/25471040; Kirsteen J. Campbell and Stephen W. C. Tait, "Targeting BCL-2 Regulated Apoptosis in Cancer," *Open Biology* 8, no. 5 (May 2018): 180002, https://doi.org/10.1098/rsob.180002, https://www.ncbi.nlm.nih.gov/pubmed/29976323; and Chien-Jui Cheng et al., "SCUBE2 Suppresses Breast Tumor Cell Poliferation and Confers a Favorable Prognosis in Invasive Breast Cancer," *Cancer Research* 69, no. 8 (April 15, 2009): 3634–41, https://doi.org/10.1158/0008-5472.CAN-08-3615, https://www.ncbi.nlm.nih.gov/pubmed/19369267.

e. Jian Zhang et al., "GSTT1, GSTP1, and GSTM1 Genetic Variants Are Associated with Survival in Previously Untreated Metastatic Breast Cancer," *Oncotarget* 8, no. 62 (December 1, 2017): 105905–14, https://doi.org/10.18632/oncotarget.22450, https://www.ncbi.nlm.nih.gov/pubmed/29285301; Emmanouil. S. Papadakis et al., "BAG-1 as a Biomarker in Early Breast Cancer Prognosis: A Systematic Review with Meta-Analyses," *British Journal of Cancer* 116, no. 12 (June 6, 2017): 1585–94, https://doi.org/10.1038/bjc.2017.130, https://www.ncbi.nlm.nih.gov/pubmed/28510570; and Chao Ni et al., "CD68- and CD163-Positive Tumor Infiltrating Macrophages in Non-metastatic Breast Cancer: A Retrospective Study and Meta-Analysis," *Journal of Cancer* 10, no. 19 (2019): 4463–72, https://doi.org/10.7150/jca.33914, https://www.ncbi.nlm.nih.gov/pubmed/31528210.

In my case, I was diagnosed with ER/PR+ HER2– invasive ductal carcinoma (IDC), somewhere between stages I and II. I had one disease-positive lymph node out of seven screened, which means I'm considered node-negative.

That one positive node still worries me, but that's an emotional rather than a rational reaction.

I had two tumors in the same breast (which may have originated from the same messed-up cell), and both were ER/PR+ HER2–. The smaller tumor was—based on Ki67 staining (remember, Ki67 helps cells divide)—growing more quickly and considered to be the more aggressive of the two, so that's the tumor we sent off for Oncotype DX testing.

My recurrence score was 21, on the low end of the intermediate-risk range. Based on the data, my five-year risk of recurrence or mortality was predicted to be 13 percent with tamoxifen (an estrogen blocker) alone versus 12 percent with tamoxifen plus chemotherapy.

So, chemo wasn't likely to help me much in terms of surviving or having the cancer come back. My medical oncologist and I agreed that I should skip chemotherapy, but he recommended that we be more aggressive with estrogen suppression since I was forty-five at the time and premenopausal (still cranking out natural estrogen). I was put into medically induced menopause (via Lupron shots), and I'm taking tamoxifen (I started out taking aromatase inhibitors but couldn't tolerate the side effects; more on that later in chapter 5). I'll likely be taking a ten-year course of tamoxifen. Since I kept my breasts, I also had a course of radiation therapy in my left breast, where the tumors were.

> *Take home:* Thanks to gene-expression profiling, I was able to avoid chemotherapy. If my Oncotype DX score had been higher and I hadn't been able to avoid chemotherapy, at least I would have had the knowledge that the chemo was actually doing me some good. Knowledge is power. If you are diagnosed with hormone receptor (ER/PR)–positive, HER2-negative early-stage breast cancer, ask for the test!

I'll touch briefly on the seventy-gene MammaPrint test,[6] since, at the time of writing, this test is less commonly used in the United States. It can be run with an eighty-gene molecular-subtyping test by the same manufacturer, called BluePrint, which gives a combined score for subtype and risk of recurrence for patients with early stage, ER+ breast cancer without positive lymph nodes up to three positive lymph nodes. Much like Oncotype DX, the MammaPrint test includes genes that regulate tumor-cell survival, insensitivity to signals that stop growth, ability to grow without pro-growth signals, limitless replicative potential (i.e., can grow indefinitely), tissue invasion and metastasis, and sustained angiogenesis (i.e., the ability to recruit blood vessels to deliver oxygen and nutrients to the tumor), along with some genes of unknown function.[7] Foundation Medicine[8] provides tests like FoundationOne CDx for solid tumors, which assesses expression of gene products for which FDA-approved drugs are available, as well as immunohistochemistry tests (e.g., staining for protein expression on thin slices of tissue from the tumor) for markers that may predict response to immune-harnessing therapy, like PD-L1 (more on that later when I talk about immune-checkpoint inhibitors in chapter 16). These tests can help your health-care team tailor a treatment plan specific to your tumor.

Surgery to Remove the Tumor(s)

Now that we've covered genomic testing, let's move on to surgery, which is part of almost all breast cancer-treatment plans. Got a tumor? It needs to go, and cutting it out is still the first, best step in treatment.

> Note: some patients are prescribed chemotherapy prior to surgery in order to shrink larger tumors. This is called *neoadjuvant chemotherapy*. For other patients with smaller tumors, chemotherapy is administered after surgery, which is called *adjuvant chemotherapy*. I'll cover chemotherapy and radiation therapies in the next chapter.

Surgical options for breast cancer currently come in two basic flavors:

- *Lumpectomy*, in which your surgeon removes the tumor, along with some surrounding tissue, preserving most of your natural breast, or

- *Mastectomy*, in which your surgeon removes your entire breast, including all of the epithelial tissue (normal and tumor), fat, and, in some cases, skin.

The mastectomy can be unilateral—or single (removal of the affected breast)—or it can be bilateral—or double (removal of both the affected and unaffected breast, or both breasts if you have bilateral breast cancer). See table 4.2 for types of surgeries and reconstruction options, with information about the pros and cons of each.

I've had two lumpectomies and a unilateral mastectomy. The first lumpectomy was to remove a benign complex papilloma from my left breast in 2016. When I was diagnosed with breast cancer in 2018, I opted for lumpectomy followed by *oncoplastic reconstruction*—a procedure that involves a breast reduction and lift. I was an excellent candidate for this option. My tumors were small, early stage, and in an anatomically accessible location for lumpectomy. Since I'm a larger, curvy woman with big breasts, the reduction maintained my proportions and created a cosmesis that worked for me (see table 4.2; and also see chapter 16, figure 16.4, for how mine looked after reconstruction). The risks included the possibility of local recurrence or residual disease, which were low, but unfortunately residual disease was an issue for me. I was aware of the risks, and I stand by my initial decision. I got unlucky, but fortunately mastectomy and follow-up reconstruction were still feasible. In February of 2020, a sharp-eyed mammography technician found a suspicious spot that turned out to be *residual disease*, which was a small bit of tumor that had likely been present but not detectable at the time of diagnosis (not to be confused with a local *recurrence*, which is when the cancer comes back in the breast some time after surgery and treatments have been completed). After my unilateral mastectomy, I opted for *autologous* (i.e., using my own tissue to build a new breast) reconstruction. I'll talk more about reconstruction in a bit.

But first, let's compare and contrast lumpectomy and mastectomy.

And before we get started, I want you to understand that there are no right or wrong choices; there are only informed choices. My goal isn't to persuade you to opt for a lumpectomy over a mastectomy, and I'm not endorsing any particular form of reconstruction. These decisions are deeply personal and as individual as each patient.

Table 4.2. Types of breast surgeries for tumor removal and reconstruction.

Breast surgery	Best candidates	Pros	Cons
Lumpectomy	Early-stage breast cancer Small tumor in an easily accessible location Not likely to create poor cosmesis	Single surgery No surgical drains	May require radiation Risk for local recurrence and residual disease
Lumpectomy plus oncoplastic reconstruction	Early-stage breast cancer Small tumor in an easily accessible location Women with larger breasts	Single surgery and reconstruction No surgical drains Pleasing cosmesis	May require radiation Risk for local recurrence and residual disease
Mastectomy	Breast cancer of any stage	Reduces risk for local recurrence No radiation required	Major surgery Surgical drains May require physical therapy for loss of mobility May require expander and delayed reconstruction
Implant reconstruction	Any	Fewer scars Works for petite/thin patients Reversible (e.g., patient can choose to change reconstruction)	Implants can break Normally need to be replaced between ten and twenty years
Autologous reconstruction	Women with more fat (donor tissue)	More natural-looking and -feeling breast Lasts a lifetime	Major surgery with drains in both breast and donor sites May require more revisions to achieve desired cosmesis
Aesthetic flat closure (form of oncoplastic reconstruction)	Any	Single surgery and reconstruction Lasts a lifetime	May require surgical drains Sometimes difficult to find and convince health-care providers to perform or honor request to perform

Note: Considerations for each type of surgery are based on tumor stage, patient body type, and personal preference. No choices are wrong. The pros and cons for each type of surgery are summarized.

A *lumpectomy* is basically a one and done if you have immediate oncoplastic reconstruction like a reduction and lift after. That's one advantage. The recovery time is also shorter, it involves no surgical drains (more on those delightful little buggers later), and, if you're like me, it's like being eighteen again with perky boobs that have cute little rosebud nipples. There's not much scar tissue, so physical therapy isn't generally necessary. The biggest drawback to lumpectomy is that, in most cases, radiation therapy is recommended after a lumpectomy to kill any residual cancer cells in the affected breast.

Radiation therapy is no joke. More on that later.

Also, prior to surgical removal of your tumor, you'll be fitted with a radar-localization device or devices, which are tiny metal reflectors that provide a signal for the detector used in the operating room so your surgeon can accurately locate the tumor. I was fitted with two SAVI SCOUT[9] devices while under mammography compression, and it involved big-ass needles that I saw go in one side of my left boob and out the other. I didn't feel it, but seeing it was pretty horrifying and jarring, especially as I was essentially trapped by the mammography machine and a large chair. (See chapter 9 for the full story.) Still, getting the needle was better than having literal *fucking wires* inserted into and sticking out of my boob before surgery, which is what they used to do prior to radar localization.[10]

With a *mastectomy*, you'll hopefully get rid of any and all cancer cells in the breast tissue, so no radiation is required. You will, however, have *surgical drains* for two to three weeks after surgery. (More on that below.) Regardless of the type of surgery you choose, your surgeon will perform a *sentinel node biopsy*. Lymph nodes serve as a collection point for fluid and cells that accumulate in tissue, recycling the fluid back into circulation and allowing immune cells in the nodes to look for signs of foreign proteins that could signal an infection. Lymph nodes in and around the breast are often the first site to which breast cancer cells spread. Prior to your mastectomy, you will receive an injection of radioactive (*Note:* it's low risk and safe) or dye tracer that the surgeon will use to locate and identify lymph nodes for biopsy. It's not fun. They give you a local anesthetic, but you're still going to feel the needle going into multiple sites along your areola. It's ouchy. But it ends quickly. And sometimes, you get a cute tech (see chapter 9).

Surgical Drains

Any time you have an injury, there's fluid and goo. Removal of one or both breasts produces a *lot* of fluid and goo. Fluid buildup inside your body after surgery is a bad thing; it can cause pain, can delay healing, and could lead to a *seroma*, which is a pocket of fluid within the surgical site that can lead to even more pain and scarring. To keep that from happening, your surgeon will place one or more hollow plastic tubes inside the surgical site, and those tubes will be attached to a soft plastic bulb that uses gentle suction to pull the fluid outside of your body.[11] The drains are held in place by a couple of stitches. You'll get at least one drain if you have a single mastectomy and up to five or six for a double mastectomy. When the bulb fills up with fluid, you or a caregiver will need to empty it and measure the amount of fluid output. As a part of your hospital discharge, you should get instructions for drain care, a cup (or cups) for measuring output, and a sheet (or sheets) to track output over time. Bring those sheets to your follow-up appointments with your surgeon so your health-care team can determine when it's okay to remove the drains. They probably won't all come out at the same time.

When emptying your drains, be sure and swab the bulb opening and cap with alcohol before you squeeze (to keep the gentle suction going) and close. This will cut down on the risk of infection. I'm not going to lie; drains suck. They're bulky and are a pain to manage when you're trying to go about your daily life, go to the bathroom, and shower/bathe/sponge bathe. And the entry sites for drains itch like a mofo! You'll have to keep them secured within special pockets in clothing designed for postmastectomy recovery, or you'll have to keep them pinned to your regular clothing. This makes dressing and undressing, bathing, and visiting the bathroom a challenge. But it's worth it to avoid the pain and complications that come with seromas.

Oh, and FYI, the stuff that drains out varies. It can be pretty red and bloody at first, but generally it gets less red and becomes clearer and honey-colored as time progresses. There will be chunks. It's shocking and gross the first time you see them, but it's perfectly normal. Better out than in!

Reconstructive Surgery

Some women can get immediate reconstruction following mastectomy if they opt for it. If you don't need radiation therapy or chemotherapy following breast removal, you may be a candidate. If you do not have immediate reconstruction, you'll be fitted with *expanders*—temporary implants placed between your chest wall and what remains of your breast skin. Their job is to preserve the shape of your skin for your future breasts. After you've recovered from the mastectomy and your surgical drains are removed, your health-care provider will begin filling the expander or expanders with saline solution each week in order to stretch your remaining skin to cover *implants* or support *autologous* tissue grafts. Your health-care provider will locate the port for injection using a magnetic device. Once the port's been located, the provider will press the location device into the skin above the port to mark it. They will then place a needle into the port—you shouldn't experience pain or much discomfort, just pressure, since mastectomy severs the nerves leading to the breast skin—and inject fifty to one hundred cubic centimeters of saline. You'll have weekly injections until the skin has been sufficiently stretched to fit the desired breast reconstruction size. Your skin will feel tight, especially near the end of the stretching process. Taking over-the-counter painkillers the day of injection can help, but please talk to your health-care team about which medications to take and which to avoid. After the final expansion, you'll need to wait four to six weeks for reconstruction, which allows the skin to rest.

Let me level with you: Expanders suck. Big time. They're uncomfortable, interfere with mobility along with scar tissue, and are just plain weird. I felt like a lopsided cyborg, even after several rounds of filling with saline (see chapter 16, figure 16.5). Plus, the expander sat much higher on my chest than my right boob, which was kind of jarring. Fortunately, I could disguise this by wearing a prosthesis in my bra. And physical therapy helped with discomfort and mobility issues. But, out of all parts of the reconstruction process, the expander was my all-time least favorite.

> A *note about reconstruction:* Breast reconstruction comes in many forms, and receiving an *aesthetic flat closure* is a perfectly acceptable choice. In a flat closure procedure—or "going flat"—the sur-

geon contours the chest wall, removing extra skin, fat, and other tissue, and tightens the remaining tissue to create a smooth, flat result. Comedian and breast cancer survivor Tig Notaro opted for flat closure.[12] Flat closure can also serve as a canvas for elaborate and beautiful tattooing.

Again, there are no right or wrong choices—only informed choices. If you opt for breast reconstruction, you can receive implants or have *autologous reconstruction*, also known as *free-flap reconstruction* (see table 4.2 for the pros and cons of each procedure.) This procedure involves transferring tissue and the arteries and veins that provide its blood supply to another part of the body—in this case, the breast. The most common form of autologous reconstruction is the *deep inferior epigastric artery perforator flap* (DIEP flap) procedure. Skin, fat, and blood vessels (but not muscle) are taken from the patient's belly and used to create a new breast. This involves microsurgical attachment of blood vessels from the flap to the blood vessels between the ribs to perfuse the flap with blood, keeping it alive. An older, less commonly utilized technique of autologous reconstruction involves taking the muscle as part of the flap; the *transverse rectus abdominis muscle flap* (TRAM flap), as it is called, does not require the microsurgery but sacrifices the muscle, which can be debilitating for the lower abdomen. If you aren't a candidate for DIEP flap, other sites that can be used for the flap include back (latissimus dorsi flap), butt (gluteal flap), and inner thigh (*transverse upper gracilis*, or TUG flap, and *diagonal upper gracilis*, or DUG flap).

Which procedure is right for you? It depends on your medical history and the size of your breasts. DIEP and TRAM flaps tend to be larger and can be used to build larger breasts. Latissimus dorsi flaps tend to work better for small to medium breasts and often require an implant (hybrid reconstruction). TUG and DUG flaps by themselves work for smaller reconstructions and are often used when a DIEP is not possible. I wasn't a candidate for DIEP because I'd had a tummy tuck before I was diagnosed with residual disease. (Hey—I'd thought I was done with cancer, and since I had nice new boobs, I'd decided to do the other half of the "mommy makeover" by getting rid of my belly fat.) In my case, my surgeon recommended a DUG flap. I'm a big, size-fourteen, curvy girl, so I had plenty of fat to spare. Complications for me came from previous radiation therapy, which had made my skin and remaining nonepithelial tissue underneath super hard and less stretchy. For many autologous procedures—as was the case for me—revisions after the first surgery that involves creating the flap may be necessary. I had to receive daily massage to loosen the hard tissue, which made it easier for my surgeon to perform the additional fat grafting that was required to plump up and smooth out the new breast (see chapter 16, figures 16.6 and 16.7 for how I looked after my DUG flap and one revision).

If you are to receive breast implants, your surgeon will remove your expanders and exchange them for either silicone or saline implants. Implants placed behind your chest muscle (pectoral muscle) require no additional support to anchor them in place. Implants placed in front of your chest muscle may require the use of additional muscle to anchor the implants, such as the latissimus muscle from your back. Basically, the muscle gets cut and wrapped around to your chest to hold the implants in place. Alternatively and more commonly in prepectoral (in front of the muscle) reconstruction, acellular dermal matrix (ADM) tissue may be used to anchor or completely wrap implants placed in front of your chest muscle. ADM is tissue that has been chemically stripped of epidermal and dermal skin cells, leaving dermal extracellular matrix behind to serve as an anchor for breast implants. The ADM is usually placed at the time the expander is placed. Depending on whether or not you have nipple- and skin-sparing mastectomy, you will likely need additional revision surgeries to construct new nipples, and/or tattooing may be used to re-create the areola—the dark area of skin around each nipple.

Choosing What's Right for You

What's the best reconstruction (or no reconstruction flat closure) choice for you? That's up to you and your health-care team. I'm not advocating lumpectomy over mastectomy or autologous reconstruction over implants. The choices I made were right for me, and other choices might be right for you. Take time to explore the pros and cons of each option (see table 4.2), and don't succumb to any pressure to decide right away. It's a big decision! You'll want time to research and, if possible, talk to breast cancer survivors who've opted for each choice that interests you. There are plenty of social media sites[13] that connect patients and survivors. In addition, several cancer organizations offer ways to connect with other patients and survivors, such as the American Cancer Society, Breastcancer.org, the National Breast Cancer Foundation, and the Cancer Support Community.[14] The breast cancer survivor community is, in my experience, open and extremely generous with sharing their advice and experiences. Your health-care team may also be able to help you connect with other patients and survivors through their center's outreach programs. Finally, make sure you are comfortable with your plastic surgeon, as they will be your guide throughout your reconstruction journey.

You might be wondering, *What are my chances of survival with a lumpectomy versus a mastectomy?* This is a great question, since keeping most of your natural breast tissue as you would with a lumpectomy comes with the risk of local recurrence (i.e., cancer coming back in the breast). Radiation therapy is often recommended with lumpectomy to mitigate that risk. You might also get unlucky like me and find residual disease (i.e., cancer that is undetectable at the time of initial diagnosis but that grows and becomes detectable later). On the other hand, mastectomy comes with a loss of sensation, since the nerves are severed when your surgeon removes the breast epithelium and fatty tissue. Surgical techniques that involve microsurgical reinnervation are being refined to partially restore sensation with autologous reconstruction, including the ongoing resensation study.[15] My awesome plastic surgeon, Dr. Galen Perdikis, is one of the study leaders.[16] Unfortunately, not every patient is a candidate for reinnervation, and many women experience persistent numbness after reconstruction.

Rates of local recurrence after lumpectomy have gone down among patients receiving "modern-era" therapies.[17] Local recurrence and residual disease can be addressed by mastectomy upon detection. That was what I chose when we found my residual disease. The gravest concern is the development of distant recurrence—or *metastasis*—where the cancer has spread to other parts of the body. The question becomes, *What is the risk for distant recurrence after lumpectomy versus mastectomy?* Turns out, the risk for distant recurrence/metastasis is the same for patients who choose lumpectomy plus radiation as it is for patients who opt for mastectomy.[18] Again, I'm not advocating for lumpectomy over mastectomy or mastectomy over lumpectomy. My goal is to arm patients with scientifically and medically vetted data that they can use to make an informed decision that is best for them.

Here are some tips for pre- and postsurgery:

1. *Start taking a stool softener before surgery.* Your health-care provider may prescribe one for you to start taking after surgery, but taking one or two doses prior can save you a lot of pain. Literally. Anesthesia can cause constipation, as can pain medications and lack of mobility. If you tend to have hard stool (like me), the first postsurgery poop can be super painful. I cried during the first one I had after autologous reconstruction. Taking stool softener the day before revision surgery really helped.

2. *Ice packs will be your friends.* Once you get the green light from your health-care provider (usually after the removal of your last surgical drain), ice packs can help reduce your pain and swelling. I've also found that they help reduce itching—not just the external stitches/surgical glue/wound closures, but also with the deep, internal itching from deep within the tissue that is so maddening because you cannot scratch it. Ice packs muted that sensation for me, along with the odd sensations that came from healing nerves. These ranged from sharp, stabbing sensations within my breasts to a strange tingling. This is a perfectly normal part of the healing process, but it's annoying at best, painful and distressing at worst.

3. *Surround yourself with pillows, bolsters, and comfy blankets.* Support is really important for comfort and safety postsurgery. Mastectomy pillows are wonderful (and also help with recovery from lumpectomy, reconstruction, and revisions). They can be heart-shaped (use one for each breast), they can be square with specially designed pockets for arm support, and there are modified versions that fit over seatbelts to keep you more comfortable while driving. For support while you sleep in your bed or in a reclining chair (it's easier to get up from a reclining chair), bolsters for under your knees, pillows to support your upper body and back (like wedge pillows), and soft, comfortable blankets can

help you rest easier and better. I'm not a natural back sleeper, and the requirement for sleeping on my back during postsurgical recovery was such a challenge. Pillows helped.

4. *Get a surgical-drain lanyard.* Postsurgical accessories include large safety pins and drainage cups for measuring output. You can pin your surgical drains to a lanyard as well as your clothing (including specialized shirts and cardigans with built-in drain pockets), but when it comes to taking a shower, a lanyard is so handy! The drains and tubes are very unwieldy, and it's really tough to hold them with one hand while you gently scrub your body with the other. A lanyard lets you go hands-free.

5. *Install a detachable showerhead.* This makes maintaining hygiene easier and will allow you to be more independent after your health-care provider says it's okay for you to start showering again after surgery. You can control water flow and where the water hits, minimizing direct contact with sutures, drainage tube inserts, and tender skin. I highly recommend installing a detachable showerhead before surgery. Using one was especially helpful after my DUG flap procedure, when I was unable to bathe due to the thigh sutures and thigh drain. And it also makes washing your hair easier when you need to protect your chest and other parts of your body.

6. *Stock up on comfortable shirts, including button-down and zip-up shirts and cotton camisoles.* After mastectomy and other procedures, you'll often be told to wait a bit before lifting your arms. When you are allowed to lift your arms, it can feel tight and painful. With button-down and zip-up shirts, you don't have to lift your arms as high. Once you get mobility back and experience less pain, soft cotton camis (especially when you're no longer wearing a compression bra) feel so good.

7. *Prepare for incision care and scar management.* Gauze or other sanitary coverings help protect your incisions and provide a cushioning barrier between your tender flesh and clothing. When I ran out of gauze, I used sanitary pads (they stick to your bra and stay in place!) and have even used soft, fuzzy socks to cushion my girls. (I'm classy like that.) When your health-care provider says it's okay, massaging the incision sites helps soften scar tissue,

which in turn helps reduce tightness and restore mobility. For cosmesis, silicone gels/gel sheets coupled with massage really help. I developed keloid scars, so the doctor who performed my tummy tuck injected steroids into the scars to help soften and flatten them, and I'll be asking Dr. Perdikis about ways we can manage my breast scars. Cosmesis is important, so don't be shy about asking your health-care team about scar management.

8. *Prioritize your mental health care.* Surgery is traumatic—not only to your body but to your mind and emotions as well. It is a stressful event for anyone and can be worse for patients living with depression and anxiety disorders. Interactions from anesthesia and antibiotics, pain, reactions to pain meds, stress related to your cancer diagnosis, and stress related to quality of life and lifespan may take a toll on your well-being.[19] Talk to your health-care team about managing the mental and emotional effects of surgery. (For more on mental, emotional, and spiritual health with breast cancer, see chapter 8.)[20]

Next up, we'll cover radiation therapy, chemotherapy, and standard-of-care molecularly targeted therapies used to treat breast cancer.

〜

CHAPTER FIVE

Radiation, Chemotherapy, and Molecularly Targeted Therapies

Weapons of Cancer Destruction

Now that we've covered tumor gene-expression-profiling tests and surgical options, let's talk about treatments, which include radiation, chemotherapy drugs, and molecularly targeted drugs. We'll start with *radiation therapy* and *chemotherapy*, treatments that target rapidly dividing cells (i.e., cells making copies of themselves quickly). Most breast cancers divide faster than cells in normal tissues, but chemotherapy and radiation can also damage and kill other rapidly dividing normal cells, like hair follicles and the cells that line your gut, which is why these treatments make patients sick and lose their hair. After that, we'll cover drugs that more specifically target breast cancer cells—*molecularly targeted therapy*—like drugs that block estrogen production and/or estrogen-receptor function, drugs that target the breast cancer oncoprotein HER2, drugs that target cyclin-dependent kinases (proteins that tell cells to divide), drugs that target VEGF (a protein produced by tumor cells that attracts blood vessels to the tumor), drugs that target the PI3K/mTOR/Akt pathway (proteins in a pathway that regulates growth and invasion), and drugs that block DNA-damage-repairing proteins.

In chapter 16 I'll give you the scoop on *immune-checkpoint inhibitors*—drugs that harness the power of a patient's own immune system to induce antitumor immunity to kill cancer cells. There we'll also cover the triumphs, the challenges, and what's on the horizon for breast cancer treatment and care, including new anti–breast cancer vaccines that have recently entered the clinical testing phase of development.

Radiation and Chemotherapy

As I mentioned in the previous chapter, *radiation therapy*—high-powered X-rays that induce DNA damage in rapidly dividing cells in the breast (including cancer cells)—is often recommended to reduce recurrence risk following a lumpectomy. How does radiation therapy work? X-rays are targeted at the area where the cancerous masses have been surgically removed, as well as the rest of the breast, and when the energy in the X-rays hits DNA, it causes double-stranded breaks. A secondary effect of the radiation is the production of *reactive oxygen species* (ROS), which also induce DNA damage, including single-stranded breaks. Breaks in DNA can be repaired, but if the damage is too extensive, the affected cells will die due to safety mechanisms that rid the body of damaged cells and tissue. Cancer cells are more prone to failed DNA-damage repair, so they are more susceptible to radiation-induced death. Remember, DNA is the blueprint for every protein needed to make a cell and allow it to perform its function. A bad blueprint makes for a nonfunctional cell. The process of damaging DNA through radiation requires time, since cancer cells need to accumulate a lot of damage; this means radiation is delivered over a course of several weeks.

For many breast cancer cases, *external-beam radiation therapy* is used. That's what I got. It involved laying on a gurney, being positioned with exquisite precision, and having the machine pointed at my left breast to deliver the beam of radiation. The machine was repositioned a couple of times during each session to zap different places. During the zapping, it's very important that you remain still and hold your breath. Inflating my lungs helped push my breast into the line of the beam while protecting my heart (definitely a concern, since I had cancer in my left breast) and lungs. This breath control is so important that they have patients practice holding their breath in advance of undergoing radiation therapy and recommend that patients do breathing exercises several times a day to make sure they can hold their breath for the twenty to thirty seconds required for each treatment zap. You'll have a dry run where they program the machine for your specific settings and simulate the treatment while you hold your breath. It feels weird, but it's important. Your health-care team wants to make certain to only hit the target area. This is because radiation doesn't just hit tumor cells; it can hit and damage cells in the entire irradiated area, hitting normal breast tissue too. So radiation therapy is tightly controlled and precisely targeted to minimize damage to normal tissue in the breast area as well as the chest wall, lung, and heart beneath the target area.[1]

As far as practical considerations go, you'll be asked to come in for daily radiation treatments five days a week, for four to six weeks, for treatment of primary breast cancer. Radiation courses may differ for treatment of metastatic breast cancer. The damage to the cancer cells and the rest of the tissue is cumulative, meaning it gets worse over time, including after treatment ends. Your breast and the surrounding area will become red and tender. The effects of treatment can be painful, and radiation therapy can cause fatigue. I was more tired than usual for about three months after my treatments ended. But there are a few things you can do to make undergoing radiation therapy easier:

1. Stock up on and wear soft cotton tank tops or camisoles.
2. Bras are a no-go on sore, burned, tender skin. Stock up on some creams to soothe your skin, and slather them on several times a day. I recommend Calendula Radiation Burn Care Cream from My Girls. I applied it just after each radiation treatment and a few more times each day, sometimes mixing with Aquaphor healing ointment.
3. Ice packs can be super soothing in the later weeks of treatment and in the weeks after treatments end. Make sure you place a soft barrier between your skin and the ice pack.
4. If you experience cracked skin, including in the area of healing incisions, definitely contact your radiation oncologist, who can prescribe topical creams to help with pain and healing.
5. Listen to your body. If you need a nap, do everything you can to make sure you can take one. I'm big on office power naps, and I went to bed early many nights after my treatments, since I was dumb/masochistic enough to keep working while undergoing radiation.

My privilege is definitely showing; some people have no *choice* but to keep working. Too many people are forced to overextend themselves to keep the bills paid while battling breast cancer. I'm a *huge* proponent of universal health care, medical leave, and other measures that will give cancer patients the security and protections they need to heal. Of course, what I *believe* won't help keep the bills paid or watch the kids, and lobbying for these measures and implementing them will take time that today's breast cancer patients don't have. If you need help, financial assistance may be available to you through Susan G. Komen's Komen Treatment Assistance Program, which offers financial assistance toward rent and utilities, transportation to and from treatment, food, child- and elder care, lymphedema care and supplies, durable medical equipment, home and palliative care, oral pain medication, anti-nausea medication, and oral chemotherapy/hormone therapy.[2] The Susan G. Komen website also provides a wealth of information, resources, and assistance obtaining health care and insurance, prescription drugs, transportation, lodging, child- and elder care, and personal expenses.[3] Other resources can be found at Cancercare.org, the Pink Fund, Metastatic Breast Cancer Network, Living Beyond Breast Cancer, and the American Breast Cancer Foundation.[4] Check for state and local resources and resources available through your medical center. Also, check into assistance with prescription medications; pharmaceutical companies sometimes have programs to help reduce costs.

Other forms of radiation therapy are sometimes used for breast cancer treatment, including *internal radiation therapy*—also called brachytherapy or *accelerated partial breast irradiation* (APBI). For this type of treatment, the radiation source is placed inside of your breast to deliver a higher radiation dose to a smaller part of the breast over a shorter amount of time. According to the American Cancer Society and BreastCancer.org, more research is needed to determine whether or not brachytherapy is as effective as whole-breast external-beam irradiation, and more careful selection criteria for patients who are good candidates for brachytherapy may need to be implemented.[5]

Next up? Chemotherapy.

Disclaimer: I have no personal experience with chemo. Thanks to a low recurrence score from my Oncotype DX test, chemotherapy wasn't recommended as a part of my treatment plan. I'll cover the science behind this type of cancer treatment, but I'll have to rely on experiences shared by friends and family to cover the practical considerations.[6]

Chemotherapy drugs in general target the process of cell division by messing around with the tumor cell's DNA blueprint or by messing around with microtubules in the cytoskeleton, interfering with the ability of dividing cells to pull apart through a process called *cytokinesis*. Figure 5.1 illustrates these modes of action for chemotherapy in cell-cycle disruption, and table 5.1 describes chemotherapy drugs used to treat breast cancer.

Cell division begins with the "mother" cell preparing for division by unwinding and replicating (making copies) of its DNA. Once the DNA is replicated, both copies line up precisely along specialized fibers from the cytoskeleton called *microtubules*, which undergo remodeling to help the DNA copies line up and separate, pulling them to opposite ends of the two, forming "daughter cells." Chemotherapy drugs work

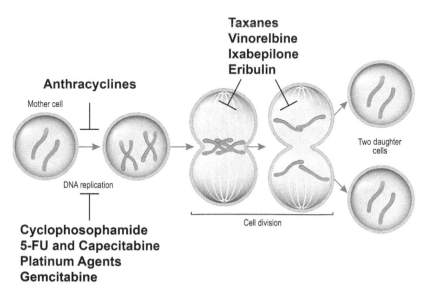

Figure 5.1. How chemotherapy disrupts cell division in rapidly dividing cells, including cancer cells. *Source:* ©iStock / ttsz.

Table 5.1. Types of chemotherapy drugs used to treat breast cancer and how they work.

Generic name(s) (Trade name[s])	Class	Mode of action	Treatment use
Doxorubicin/adriamycin (Lipodox, Lipodox 50, Doxil*)	Anthracycline	Intercalates (i.e., wedges itself between base pairs) into DNA and RNA, causing damage	Neoadjuvant/adjuvant therapy; metastatic disease * Note: Liposomal formulations of doxorubicin used in metastatic disease, neoadjuvant therapy
Epirubicin (Ellence)	Anthracycline	Intercalates (i.e., wedges itself between base pairs) into DNA and RNA, causing damage	Neoadjuvant/adjuvant therapy; metastatic disease
Cyclophosphamide (Cytoxan or Neosar)	Alkylating agent	Binds to DNA and RNA, causing damage and blocking DNA replication and protein translation from mRNA	Neoadjuvant/adjuvant therapy
Paclitaxel/abraxane+ (Taxol)	Taxane	Interferes with microtubule reorganization during cell division	Neoadjuvant/adjuvant therapy; metastatic disease + Note: Albumin-encapsulated form
Docetaxel (Docefrez and Taxotere)	Taxane	Interferes with microtubule reorganization during cell division	Neoadjuvant/adjuvant therapy; metastatic disease
5-fluorouracil (5-FU) (Fluoroplex, Tolak, Efudex, Carac, and Adrucil)	Antimetabolite	Mimics nucleotides in DNA and RNA, blocking DNA replication and protein translation from mRNA	Neoadjuvant/adjuvant therapy

Drug	Class	Mechanism	Use
Capecitabine (Xeloda)	Antimetabolite	Mimics nucleotides in DNA and RNA, blocking DNA replication and protein translation from mRNA	Adjuvant therapy; also metastatic disease
Gemcitabine (Gemzar)	Antimetabolite	Mimics nucleotides in DNA, blocking DNA replication	Metastatic disease
Carboplatin (Paraplatin)	Platinum agent	Binds to DNA and causes damage, preventing DNA replication	Neoadjuvant/adjuvant therapy; metastatic disease
Cisplatin (Platinol)	Platinum agent	Binds to DNA and causes damage, preventing DNA replication	Neoadjuvant/adjuvant therapy; metastatic disease
Vinorelbine (Navelbine)	Plant alkaloid	Interferes with microtubule reorganization during cell division	Metastatic disease
Ixabepilone (Ixempra)	Antimicrotubule agent	Interferes with microtubule reorganization during cell division	Metastatic disease
Eribulin (Halaven)	Halichondrine	Interferes with microtubule reorganization during cell division	Second line in advanced cancers

Note: *Neoadjuvant* (used before surgery) and *adjuvant* (used after surgery) drugs are often used in combinations of two to three drugs. Chemotherapies are normally used as single agents rather than in combination for patients with metastatic disease that has spread outside the breast and underarm area, either at the time of diagnosis or after initial treatments.

by either disrupting DNA replication or by interfering with microtubule remodeling. Since most tumor cells divide more rapidly than the cells around them, they are more susceptible to chemotherapy-induced DNA damage and chemotherapy-induced disruption of daughter-cell separation. Unfortunately, other rapidly dividing cells in the patient's body get hit as collateral damage. (More on that later.) Some of the ways chemotherapy works include

1. Inducing DNA damage (like radiation), or mimicking the building blocks of DNA and RNA. If the fake building blocks get put in place of the real nucleotide building blocks, then DNA replication (copy machine) and mRNA translation to protein (reading the three-letter code for each amino acid) can't work.
2. Interfering with DNA copying (replication), inhibiting separation of DNA strands necessary for DNA replication.
3. Inhibiting mitosis, the process of cell division.

These all result in cell death.

Chemotherapy can be administered directly into the patient's bloodstream by intravenous infusion or through a port that has been surgically implanted and connects to a large vein. This port can also be used to collect blood for testing throughout the treatment course. Some chemotherapies are injected into muscle or fat. Other chemotherapies drugs can be taken in pill form.[7] See table 5.1 for common chemotherapy and how these drugs work.

Unlike radiation therapy, chemotherapy is a *systemic therapy*—meaning the drug travels throughout a patient's body. It doesn't specifically attack tumor cells, just cells that divide quickly—which is why chemotherapy has such nasty side effects. Hair follicles, blood and immune cells, and the cells lining gut tissue (stomach and intestines) all divide rapidly; this means they are caught in the crossfire of chemotherapy and cancer cells, and chemotherapy can produce side effects like hair loss, anemia, immune-system compromise, nausea, and diarrhea.[8] Additional side effects can include the following:

1. *Neuropathy*, caused by the effects of chemotherapy on nerve endings in hands and feet, can lead to pain, numbness and/or tingling and burning sensations, increased sensitivity to cold and heat, and weakness in extremities. Neuropathy can go away within a year or more after finishing chemotherapy, or can last longer.
2. *Chemo brain* refers to the neurologic and cognitive side effects that chemotherapy causes by affecting the brain, including problems with short-term memory; difficulty remembering names and dates or finding words; difficulty concentrating; and taking longer than usual to finish tasks. Chemo brain is a serious issue, especially since these effects can persist in patients long after chemotherapy is complete.

Note that, according to the American Cancer Society, symptoms similar to chemo brain can also crop up in patients after cancer surgery and radiation, as well as in some patients treated with hormone blockers.[9] Other factors that can contribute to cognitive difficulties related to cancer therapy include other medications (including anesthesia used during surgery), other health conditions like diabetes and high blood pressure, being tired and having sleep problems, pain, mental-health issues like anxiety and depression, age, being postmenopausal or undergoing hormone changes or treatments, infection, weakness or frailty, malnutrition, and alcohol and drug use.

I can personally attest to brain fog and cognitive issues resulting from hormone blockers, especially aromatase inhibitors (AIs). Tamoxifen hasn't been as bad for me, though I still struggle finding the right word or finishing a thought on occasion. I noticed changes when I took exemestane (Aromasin, an aromatase inhibitor; more on this drug later on). My spelling went to hell, as did my ability to write coherently. It was frightening, especially for someone who makes a living with her brain and for whom writing is a passion. Every patient is unique, and not everyone will have the same response to specific drugs or experience all possible side effects. My best advice is to talk to your health-care team about changes you notice in mental function.

What can you do to help fight chemo brain and brain fog during your breast cancer treatment? Ask your health-care team about *cognitive-rehabilitation programs* available at your cancer center or medical center. These programs are designed to help with brain function, "exercising" the brain by having you performing activities that become harder over time to build a stronger brain, and they help you learn new ways to process information, try new tasks, and use organizational tools such as diaries and planners. Physical exercise helps too and is just all-around good for your body and mind. Even simple activities like gardening, walking, or taking care of pets (pets are wonderful—my cats gave me special attention, healing purrs, and TLC after each surgery and during radiation treatments) can help with mental function. Meditation can do the same. My personal go-to is yoga, which is a great way to combine physical activity with meditation. Believe me, it's impossible to let your mind wander while concentrating on not falling on your ass while holding a yoga pose.

I know a lot of you are rolling your eyes because you've been asked, "Have you tried yoga??" one too many times. But I actually found it helpful. Yoga practice at home at least three times a week has been a game changer for me. Yoga with Adriene is my personal favorite; she got me through COVID-19 lockdown and kept me fit and sane prior to mastectomy and reconstruction surgeries.[10] But maybe there is something else you prefer—barre exercise? Pilates? Long walks with a friend, spouse, child, pet, or yourself? Pedicures? Find something that works for you, your body, and your state of mind during treatments.

I know several of you are thinking, "Exercise? *During chemotherapy?* Are you fucking kidding me??"

Okay, hear me out. You don't have to run sprints or marathons or break yourself while you're in pain and fatigued; I wouldn't recommend that for anyone. But on those days between chemo infusions when you're feeling okay enough to get up and walk, do a little gardening (sunshine and fresh air), have a swim, or do a little light, low-impact yoga that focuses more on body/mind connection and meditation rather than intense poses. Give it a try. It goes back to one of my favorite tools (seriously, I have it taped to my door at home and at the office): "Everything Is Awful and I'm Not Okay: Questions to Ask before Giving Up"—a series of questions to ask yourself to help manage discomfort and distress.[11] Have you stretched your legs some time in the past day? Have you moved your body to music in the past twenty-four hours? Dancing around the house in your underwear is great exercise—good for the mood, the mind, and the soul. (Just make sure your blinds are closed; I think I gave my neighbors a show they never wanted to see not long ago . . .[12])Whatever it is that works for you, try to fit in at least some moderate exercise and a bit of time outside every day. Your body and mind will thank you for it.

As I've already mentioned, hair loss as a side effect of chemotherapy occurs because the drugs used target rapidly growing cells, which include hair follicles. This means *all* hair follicles—eyebrows, eyelashes, pubes. My cousin Sherri said that when she went through chemotherapy, it was like being eight years old all over again. The hair loss is reversible, but the hair that grows back may be different in texture than your prechemo hair. Anemia and immune-system compromise come from the effect of chemotherapy on rapidly growing progenitor cells in the bone marrow (e.g., cells that have the potential to become mature red blood cells and immune cells); this might make patients feel tired and more prone to infections. These side effects are also reversible.

Hormone Therapy

Other anticancer drugs are more specific than chemotherapy. A large class of selective estrogen receptor modulators (SERMs)—drugs that can either activate or block estrogen-receptor function—are used to treat ER+ breast cancers, which account for about 80 percent of all breast cancers.[13] In the case of breast cancer, SERMs act as *antagonists*—which means they block ER function. Drugs that block estrogen synthesis—called *aromatase inhibitors* (AIs)—are also used for ER+ breast cancer, often in conjunction with induction of menopause in premenopausal patients through removal of ovaries or by using drugs to suppress ovarian function. In my case, I receive shots of leuprolide acetate (trade name Lupron) every three months to maintain medically induced menopause. The drug works by blocking secretion of the hormone gonadotropin, which in turn stops my ovaries from producing estrogen.[14] SERMs come in pill form.

Before we go on, let's cover what estrogen does in normal breast tissue and how it gets roped into helping breast cancer cells grow. *Estrogen is a sex-specific hormone, produced mostly by ovaries, that circulates through a biologically female body starting at puberty.* Among other things, estrogen stimulates breast epithelial cells to grow; that's why your breasts may feel lumpy and sore just before your menstrual cycle. The glands are growing and getting geared up in case of pregnancy so they can start the process of differentiation to a milk-production and -delivery factory (see chapter 1). At the molecular level, the hormone estrogen enters a cell and binds to estrogen receptors—proteins that function as *transcription factors*. Transcription factors go to the nucleus of cells and bind DNA, regulating the transcription of mRNA, which will then be translated to proteins. The estrogen/estrogen receptor causes cells to make mRNA-encoding proteins that make breast cells grow, like cell-cycle regulators that drive cell division. In breast cancer, high levels of estrogen-receptor proteins make cells grow super fast.

Some SERMs used to treat breast cancer include tamoxifen (the first estrogen blocker developed for treating breast cancer; trade name Novadex), toremifene (trade name Fareston), and lasofoxifene (trade name Fablyn), which is being tested for effectiveness in ER+ breast cancer patients with a mutation in estrogen receptor 1, ESR1.[15] Another antiestrogen drug that works by blocking or damaging estrogen receptors is fulvestrant (trade name Faslodex), classified as a *selective estrogen receptor degrader* (SERD). It is most commonly used to treat advanced breast cancer, including breast cancers that have stopped responding to other hormone blockers, and metastatic breast cancer in combination with other drugs. It is administered as an injection. As renowned medical oncologist Dr. Ben Ho Park told me, fulvestrant "is literally a pain in the butt—actually, two pains in the butt, since we give two injections."

Aromatase inhibitors (AIs) include letrozole (trade name Femara), anastrozole (trade name Arimidex), and exemestane (trade name Aromasin). They come in pill form, and they're normally used to treat postmenopausal women with breast cancer, though these drugs can be used in premenopausal women in combination with ovarian-suppression therapy.[16] Aromatase is an *enzyme*—a protein that performs chemical reactions in the body. Aromatase is part of the metabolic pathway that your body uses to make estrogen, so drugs that inhibit this enzyme's function stop your body from making estrogen and help stop ER+ breast cancer cells from growing.

What are the side effects of these drugs? With SERMS, if you aren't already in menopause, you may experience some of the not-so-fun effects of lowered hormone levels, including hot flashes, night sweats, and fatigue, as well as vaginal dryness and sexual dysfunction (more on that coming up in chapter 14). Other less common but more serious side effects may include increased risk for uterine cancer in postmenopausal women, which is why you should definitely keep up with your annual gynecologic screenings, and vascular side effects including blood clots. Deep vein thrombosis and pulmonary embolism are life-threatening, so contact your health-care providers immediately if you experience swelling or pain in your legs or chest pain and shortness of breath.

Fulvestrant and AIs also produce menopause-like symptoms. While AIs don't put patients at risk for uterine cancer or at high risk for blood clots, they do often cause pain in muscles and joints. I experienced these side effects when I tried letrozole and later when I switched to exemestane. Over the course of eight months on letrozole, my fatigue and pain levels gradually increased to the point where I had a hard time physically getting out of bed, getting into and out of my car, and moving around generally. AIs also increase bone thinning, putting patients at risk for osteoporosis and bone breaks. This is because estrogen also functions to maintain bone building. Ask your health-care team about periodic screenings for changes in bone density while you're taking AIs.

Which estrogen-suppression strategy is right for you? Again, it depends on whether you're pre- or postmenopausal, the stage of your breast cancer, and whether you've been treated with other estrogen blockers that have stopped working. Your medical oncologist will recommend a treatment strategy based on the latest scientific and clinical data available to keep your cancer at bay. But determining a treatment plan is not an exact science. Every patient's physiology and cancer biology are unique, and how you respond to specific estrogen blockers and their effects on your quality of life should factor into the equation too. Communication is key. For example, if your hot flashes and night sweats are out of control on one type of medication, talk to your oncologist about how to fight those side effects or about whether trying another medication would be better. The same goes for other side effects, including joint and muscle pain, fatigue, brain fog, and the sexual side effects that we don't talk about enough (more on that in chapter 14).

HER2-Targeted Therapies

For HER2+ breast cancers—which are driven by a cell-surface protein receptor that tells cells to grow uncontrollably when amplified or dysregulated—molecularly targeted anti-HER2 inhibitors like trastuzumab (trade name Herceptin), pertuzumab (trade name Perjeta), and margetuximab (trade name Margenza), which are monoclonal antibody therapies, and tucatinib (Tukysa), which are kinase inhibitors, have revolutionized treatment of this aggressive breast cancer subtype that represents 20 to 25 percent of all breast cancers. For more on the development and history of Herceptin, I recommend Robert Bazell's *Her-2: The Making of Herceptin, a Revolutionary Treatment for Breast Cancer*.[17] It's one hell of a story full of the drama and politics of academia, medicine, and pharma and biotech corporate culture, the power of advocacy in the fight for compassionate use, and the very human story of the patients who paved the way for this remarkable treatment by volunteering for clinical trials.

Prior to the development of Herceptin, the prognosis for HER2+ breast cancer was grim, with high rates of recurrence and progression to metastatic disease. Today Herceptin and other HER2-inhibitors have improved four-year survival rates for HER2+ disease, with survival rates of 82.7 percent for hormone receptor–negative HER2+ disease and 90.3 percent for hormone receptor–positive HER2+ disease.[18] These statistics reflect patients diagnosed with early-stage disease that has not spread beyond regional lymph nodes. HER2+ breast cancer patients are usually treated with chemotherapy as well as anti-HER2 therapies.

How do these drugs work? Monoclonal antibody therapies like Herceptin work like the antibodies your own body produces in response to an infection. They "tag" cells expressing HER2 protein and target them for destruction by your immune system. These therapies are delivered by infusion into the patient's bloodstream through a slow-drip intravenous infusion or by subcutaneous (e.g., beneath the skin) injection, anywhere from once a week to once every three weeks, for a year or more after diagnosis, depending on disease stage at diagnosis.[19] Versions of these therapies called *antibody drug conjugates* (ADCs), in which the antibody is attached to another cancer-fighting drug, are also used to treat certain types of HER2+ breast cancer (e.g., ado-trastuzumab, fam-trastuzumab deruxtecan). Kinase inhibitors like lapatinib bind to the active part of the HER2 protein, the kinase domain, and to stop the protein from sending signals to the cancer cells that tell them to grow. These drugs are available in pill form.

What are the side effects of HER2-targeted therapies? Aside from severe diarrhea and hand-foot syndrome (soreness and reddening of hands and feet, which can lead to blistering and peeling), these drugs can cause damage to the heart, and the risk is higher if used in combination with certain chemotherapy drugs like doxorubicin (trade name Adriamycin) and epirubicin (trade name Ellence). Your health-care team should monitor your heart function before and during treatment. Definitely contact your health-care team right away if your legs swell, if you experience shortness of breath, or if you become really fatigued.

Other Targeted Therapies

A class of drugs that inhibit proteins regulating cell cycle—the process through which cells divide and become uncontrolled in cancers—has emerged in the past decade. These cyclin-dependent kinase (CDK) inhibitors work by inactivating proteins called cyclin-dependent kinases, which serve as a "go" signal for cell division. Current FDA-approved CDK inhibitors include palbociclib (trade name Ibrance), ribociclib (trade name Kisqali), and abemaciclib (trade name Verzenio) and are often used in combination with AIs or fulvestrant in advanced ER+ breast cancers. Side effects patients might experience include fatigue and low blood counts, which could put patients at risk for infection. CDK inhibitors come in pill form.

Everolimus (trade name Afinitor) blocks the function of a kinase called mTOR that regulates growth and metabolism and also helps cancers attract new blood vessels. This drug is used in postmenopausal patients with advanced ER+ breast cancer and may be combined with the AI exemestane in patients with cancers that have grown while being treated with either letrozole or anastrozole AIs or in cases where the cancer started growing shortly after treatment with these AIs was stopped. Side effects may include mouth sores, diarrhea, nausea, fatigue, low blood counts, shortness of breath, and cough. Everolimus can also make blood cholesterol, triglycerides, and blood sugar levels go up. Your health-care team will check your blood for these possible side effects while you're on this medication. It comes in pill form.

Speaking of blood, breast tumors can attract new blood vessels to feed and sustain them. One way they do that is by producing a secreted protein called *vascular endothelial growth factor* (VEGF). Like all rapidly growing tissues in your body, cancer needs oxygen and nutrition to survive. Tumor blood vessels also help tumors grow bigger and spread. Cancers get this blood supply by tricking your body into sending new blood-vessel sprouts to perfuse the tumor, a process known as *angiogenesis*. Making and sending out VEGF protein is a major mechanism tumors use to trick the body into growing new blood vessels, and a drug called bevacizmab (trade name Avastin) stops VEGF from reaching and communicating with proteins on the surface of blood vessels that respond to VEGF. Like Herceptin, bevacizumab is an antibody therapy, binding to and blocking VEGF, and it can be used as part of the treatment plan for patients with metastatic breast cancer in combination with chemotherapy. Side effects may include high blood pressure, nose bleeds, weakness, pain, and diarrhea, and less common but more serious side effects include blood clots and related complications. Just like with SERMs, you should contact your health-care team immediately if you experience swelling or pain in your legs or chest pain and shortness of breath while on bevacizumab. This drug is delivered by intravenous infusion.

Alpelisib (trade name Piqray) is another drug that can be used in combination with fulvestrant to treat postmenopausal women with advanced hormone receptor–positive, HER2-negative breast cancer with a *PIK3CA* gene mutation and with cancer that has grown during or after treatment with an AI. Alpelisib works by stopping the activity of the PI3K protein, which causes breast cancer cells to grow uncontrollably. The *PIK3CA* mutation makes PI3K more active, which gives the tumor a growth advantage; around 30 to 40 percent of breast cancers have this mutation. The drawbacks with this drug are a long list of side effects that include high blood-sugar levels; kidney, liver, and pancreatic problems; diarrhea; low blood counts; nausea and vomiting; fatigue; decreased appetite; mouth sores; weight loss; low calcium levels; blood-clotting problems; and hair loss. Rashes—even severe rashes that result in skin peeling and blistering—are possible. Alpelisib comes in pill form.

For patients with mutations in BRCA genes—either carriers of familial mutations (hereditary breast cancer) or mutations that form spontaneously in tumors—drugs called PARP inhibitors can be used. PARP inhibitors like olaparib (trade name Lynparza) and talazoparib (trade name Talzenna) work by stopping the protein PARP from repairing damaged DNA in cancer cells. Since BRCA mutations already result in more DNA damage, blocking repair sets the cell up to die. These drugs are used for metastatic HER2– breast cancers that have already been treated with chemotherapy and in hormone receptor–positive breast cancers that have been treated with hormone therapy so long as these cancers carry a BRCA mutation. According to Dr. Ben Ho Park—medical oncologist quoted above—results from the phase-3 adjuvant-therapy trial are going to be announced soon, and recent press releases report positive results.[20] Side effects might include nausea and vomiting, diarrhea, fatigue, reduced appetite, changes in taste, anemia, low platelet and white blood-cell counts, belly pain, and muscle and joint pain. PARP inhibitors come in pill form.

Last but not least, in April 2020, the FDA granted accelerated approval for the first molecularly targeted therapy for the triple-negative breast cancer subtype.[21] Sacituzumab govitecan (trade name Trodelvy) targets Trop-2—a specific protein that breast cancer cells overproduce and that causes cancer cells to grow quickly and spread. This drug is an ADC (antibody drug conjugate): the antibody part binds to Trop-2, delivering chemotherapy (drug conjugate) to the cancer cells that make too much Trop-2 to kill them. Sacituzumab govitecan has been approved for metastatic triple-negative breast cancers that have failed to respond to standard chemotherapy and is delivered by intravenous infusion. Patients normally get a dose of meds to stop allergic reactions before getting Trodelvy. Side effects can include nausea and vomiting, diarrhea, constipation, fatigue, rash, lowered appetite, hair loss, anemia, and belly pain.

All of these therapies come with the risk of infertility, which is a serious consideration for younger women diagnosed with breast cancer.[22]

Even more therapies to treat breast cancer are in the pipeline in the laboratory and in clinical trials. The most urgent unmet need is for drugs to help patients with triple-negative breast cancer and patients with metastatic disease. Immune-checkpoint inhibitors have the potential to help patients with these types of cancer, as do breast cancer vaccines that have recently entered clinical trials. Currently, abraxane and immune-checkpoint inhibitor atezolizumab have been approved for treatment of metastatic triple-negative breast cancers that are 1 percent positive for PDL1-checkpoint inhibitor ligand. I'll cover those in chapter 16, as well as some work that my laboratory has been doing to see if targeting the EphA2 cell-surface protein kinase can help with HER2+, triple-negative, and metastatic breast cancer in chapter 13.

But first we need to talk about privilege and disparities.

This discussion is not only relevant to people who face extra challenges when it comes to cancer care; it is also important for people who enjoy racial, social, and economic privilege to know what's going on. It is crucial that we *all* understand what people of color, LGBTQIA+[23] folks, poor people, and disabled or differently abled people face in the health-care system—assuming they have access at all, which isn't always the case—if we are going to create equality and equity in cancer care. And we *should* work for equality and equity in cancer care. It's the right thing to do. Breast cancer already sucks enough without disparities making it worse.

I'll cover disparities in the next chapter. Read on.

CHAPTER SIX

~

Cancer Doesn't Discriminate, But We Do

Disparities and Cancer

This chapter by no means provides a comprehensive discussion of disparities in health care or even cancer care in particular. There are entire fields of research dedicated to this topic; I've barely scratched the surface. But I would be doing readers a huge disservice by failing to acknowledge the issues faced by racial and ethnic minorities, the LGBTQIA+ community, and people with disabilities. I've always been aware on some level that disparities in care exist, but it wasn't until I participated in a collaborative project with the Middle Tennessee Affiliate of the Susan G. Komen organization[1] in 2012 that I began to truly understand the scope of the issue. My colleague, longtime collaborator, and dear friend Dr. Rebecca Cook was approached by the affiliate chapter to help them apply to the parent organization for money to use for programs in middle Tennessee. To do that, they first needed to identify areas with a high prevalence of breast cancer and higher mortality rates. Using this information, they could figure out what interventions Komen could implement to support the unique needs of the diverse population in middle Tennessee. When Rebecca approached me, I took advantage of my institution's support for clinical research and received funding for statistical support in interrogating cancer data curated by the Surveillance, Epidemiology, and End Results (SEER) Program.[2] The goal was to look at breast cancer incidence and mortality throughout the affiliate service area—a mixture of urban, suburban, and rural, affluent and impoverished, and de facto racially segregated communities.

The results were eye-opening for me; our data analysis highlighted disparities in cancer incidence and mortality related to race, income, insurance coverage, mammography-screening rates that may be due to lack of access due to geographic or financial restrictions, and socio-economic status.[3] Williamson County is definitely "the land of milk and honey," as my colleague Rebecca so aptly put it, with its largely White, affluent, well-educated, and well-insured population. Since participating in this research, I've developed a keen interest in dispari-ties when it comes to breast cancer in the laboratory, such as a focus on identification and preclinical validation of a new molecular target for triple-negative breast cancer, a subtype that disproportionately af-fects Black women.[4] This has also influenced my work in advocacy and outreach—a new role I've been pursing since my personal adventure with breast cancer—including this book chapter.

As a middle-class, cis-heterosexual, able-bodied, neurotypical White woman with stable financial resources, health insurance, and access to state-of-the-art health care—plus access to a health-care system that doesn't make me feel uncomfortable or unwelcome except where it's actually rooted in benevolent sexism—I hit the jackpot, and it shows. My cancer was diagnosed early thanks to access to and coverage for routine preventative care. I live in a city with lots of hospitals, clinics, and medical centers, and I have reliable transportation that allowed me to easily travel to and from my appointments. I have a fairly cushy, flexible job in academia that includes paid medical leave, which I took advantage of to recover from each surgery; I didn't and don't have to worry about being fired because of all the extra time I've spent going to follow-up appointments.

I didn't have to choose between taking my meds and paying my mortgage. I didn't have to worry about putting food on the table for my family because my cancer treatments cost too much.

I didn't have to start a GoFundMe to cover the costs of my care.

Seriously, in 2019 one-third of all GoFundMe donations went to cover medical expenses.[5] No one should have to crowdfund to live. Yet too many Americans do have to worry about those things. A cancer diagnosis leads to financial ruin for too many families in the United States or to unnecessary pain, suffering, and death for others who are diagnosed late and cannot afford proper treatment. Why? It's complicated and involves many factors, including

1. A rise in the cost of cancer care related to an increasingly aging population (age is still a top risk factor for all cancers, including breast)
2. The trend toward treating patients with more anticancer therapies in combination for a longer time period
3. The increasing costs of advanced diagnostic tools and imaging
4. And the high costs of cancer drugs, which includes a price tag of over $100,000 for over half of newly approved drugs.[6]

And, of course, there's the lack of health insurance or inadequate health insurance, which results in a 60 percent increase in the likelihood of death from breast cancer.[7]

If you're lucky enough to even have health insurance, you may still face astronomical costs for care due to increases in deductibles, copays, and coinsurance rates. If you don't have health insurance, either you bear the burden of these exorbitant expenses on your own, or you forgo treatment and risk your life. Cancer also creates a vicious cycle of financial peril due to lost income, since cancer treatments require significant time off work, and many jobs do not offer paid medical leave. In fact, according to Yabroff et al., "Health care for illness and related income losses because of employment changes as a result of illness are a leading cause of personal bankruptcy, especially for cancer survivors." A systematic review of published literature found that people who experienced a disruption in health-insurance coverage or were underinsured were less likely to get preventative cancer screenings, more likely to have advanced disease when diagnosed, less likely to receive necessary treatments, and more likely to die.[8] Uninsured women were 2.6 times more likely to be diagnosed with breast cancer at a late stage than women with insurance, and five-year survival rates for women without insurance or with Medicaid were lower than for women with private or other insurance.[9]

So maybe the United States should, I don't know, provide universal health-care coverage like every other industrialized nation on the planet?? It would help.

But expanding coverage is only one piece of the puzzle that is improving outcomes and eliminating disparities for breast cancer patients. As noted in an article highlighting the findings of the European Society for Medical Oncology Congress, the issue is complex, and having a national health-care system does not guarantee access to cancer care.[10] Many European health-care systems face the same challenges with drug costs that plague the United States' health-care system, and some systems have lengthy processes for addition of new drugs eligible for coverage or reimbursement. Differences in early cancer-diagnosis rates result in lower survival in nations like Denmark, England, Northern Ireland, and Wales compared to survival rates in Australia, Canada, and Sweden. And in the United States, simply expanding insurance coverage won't eliminate racial disparities in breast cancer outcomes, as a recent study reported that differences in health insurance only accounted for 35 percent of the increased risk of breast cancer death between Black women and White women.[11]

So, what else is going on?

Spoiler alert: It's systemic racism.

Black women face many barriers related to race when it comes to health care in general and breast cancer care in particular, compounded by pervasive sexism within the US health-care system, resulting in stress when approaching health care. Even college-educated former CDC employees have to sell themselves as "credible witnesses," like Dr. Tina Sacks, who goes so far as to wear her CDC badge to appointments just to get her health-care providers to take her seriously.[12] Dr. Sacks details experiences faced by middle-class Black patients in her book *Invisible Visits: Black Middle-Class Women in the American Healthcare System*, which I highly recommend for more insight into higher infant mortality rates, racial profiling, and racist attitudes when it comes to pain management for Black patients and their struggle to have health-care concerns taken seriously by providers.[13]

In addition to facing bias from health-care providers, the Black community persistently encounters trust issues when it comes to health care/cancer care and participation in clinical trials.[14] Black bodies have long been exploited in the name of "research." From the infamous and cruel gynecological "studies" Dr. James Marion Sims conducted on enslaved Black women without their consent (or anesthesia)[15] to the Tuskegee Study that tracked disease progression of Black men with syphilis without treatment[16] even when treatment had became available (the study participants were lied to, told they had received proper treatment), the development of HeLa cells without the knowledge or consent of Henrietta Lacks, whose family still struggles financially and in terms of health-care access,[17] and other horrors, Black people in the United States have a history of facing medical abuse and have every right to question if their (largely White) health-care providers have their best interests at heart. Past abuses aside, what we need to focus on today is dismantling the institutional racism that Black women experience in the health-care setting today, from dismissiveness to neglect to improper pain management.

Indeed, it is important to note that surveys of Black Americans have found that wariness about participating in research was not associated with Tuskegee, and efforts by clinicians and scientists to enroll Black patients in clinical studies are woefully lacking, highlighting issues with modern-day barriers to health-care service for Black patients. Dr. Karen Lincoln, associate professor of social work and senior scientist at the University of Southern California's Suzanne Dworak-Peck School of Social Work, says that blaming Tuskegee for underrepresentation of Black Americans in medical trials is "an excuse. If you continue to use it as a way of explaining why many African Americans are hesitant, it almost absolves you of having to learn more, do more, involve other people—admit that racism is actually a thing today."[18]

Breast cancer survivor and comedian Wanda Sykes points out in her Netflix special *Wanda Sykes: Not Normal*, that health-care providers are more likely to prescribe opioids to White patients than Black patients—a result of the racist notion that Black people aren't as sensitive to pain as Whites.[19] After Wanda's double mastectomy, she was sent home with Ibuprofen. I got opioids.

Similar discrimination and resulting mistrust exist for Hispanic and Latinx people, with some overlapping factors like systemic racism, poverty, and lack of health insurance to blame, as well as unique challenges for Hispanic patients, like lack of culturally appropriate health services, including providers who speak Spanish, and the issue of immigration status. Like Black patients, Hispanic patients as well as Indigenous and Alaska Native patients are at the time of diagnosis more disproportionately diagnosed with more advanced breast cancers, have limited access to high-quality cancer care, and have higher incidences of triple-negative breast cancer, a particularly aggressive breast cancer subtype for which treatment options are limited. Other overlapping factors that affect breast cancer incidence and outcome disparities in Black and Hispanic women include comorbidities like type 2 diabetes and obesity, the rates of which are higher for these women of color than they are for White women. Women of color are also more likely to live in poor areas plagued with elevated exposure to environmental pollution.[20]

Because of systemic racism and its impacts on our medical and scientific institutions, and because of the lack of trust people of color have in clinical research and health-care settings, people of color are less represented in clinical studies and clinical trials. When it comes to identifying unique genetic mutations that may be more prevalent in different racial or ethnic groups due to ancestry, we definitely face the problem of underrepresentation. Most gene-expression data linked to clinical outcomes has been derived from studies that include mostly White people.[21]

> This means we're missing information that could improve screening for relevant mutations and alterations associated with specific ethnic groups that may contribute to disease, as well as missing opportunities for therapies that could improve outcomes.

Genome-wide association studies (GWAS)—which analyze genomes from lots and lots of people to look for genetic markers that may predict the presence of a disease—have recently identified new genetic loci (i.e., locations on DNA) associated with breast cancer in East Asian populations, a susceptibility locus for hormone receptor–negative breast cancer in Black women, and a genetic variant associated with a lower risk for breast cancers, including hormone receptor–negative breast cancer, in Hispanic women.[22] There are probably more such mutations and new gene variants to be discovered, and finding them could save lives. The medical and scientific community needs to work hard to establish trust with historically underserved and abused groups so that we can better serve *all* cancer patients.

LGBT/LGBTQIA+ patients face overlapping and unique challenges and disparities when it comes to cancer care.

> These barriers and the ways to overcome them have not been as well studied as have disparities based solely on poverty (socioeconomic status), race, and ethnicity.[23]

Smoking and alcohol consumption increase cancer risk, and rates of these behaviors are higher in LGBT youth.[24] LGBT people tend to be disproportionately poor and uninsured relative to cis-heterosexual people in the United States, though the Affordable Care Act (ACA) has reduced the number of uninsured. Moreover, mandates associated with the ACA require coverage for sex-specific recommended preventive services for people whose "gender identity or recorded gender is not in concordance with the sex-specific service."[25] That means that trans men qualify for mammography screening and pap smears, which are essential for early detection of breast and cervical cancer. Having universal health-care coverage and protections for marginalized populations helps! These provisions have been (unnecessarily) politicized and are still under attack. We need to protect and expand them.

By the way, don't @ me with the whole "what about my religious freedom—my god tells me being gay is a sin" bullshit. If you choose to work in health care, you choose to provide care for *all* patients. There's an oath and everything—you know, first do no harm? Denying care based on prejudice does lots of harm. If you're too bigoted to provide care to people who aren't like you, you can and should find another profession. Period.

Speaking of prejudice, because of it, many gay people are uncomfortable disclosing their sexual orientation out of fear that the disclosure might negatively impact their health-care providers' attitude toward them, including denial of care.[26] LGBT-specific health-care providers have documented derogatory comments, disrespect, and discrimination that LGBT patients and their partners face.[27] This treatment definitely affects quality of care and (un)willingness of gay people to seek care in the first place. For trans patients who cannot avoid disclosure of their trans identity in the health-care setting, lack of trust and gaps in knowledge about trans health are significant barriers to seeking care and finding care, including cancer care.

One important question regarding the trans community: *Are trans individuals at increased risk of breast cancer?* After all, a cis woman's breast cancer risk is related to exposure to estrogen and progesterone produced by her ovaries. Longer exposure times to hormones due to early menarche (younger age at first period), late menopause, and later age of first pregnancy or no lifetime pregnancy history all increase the risk,[28] as well as *hormone replacement therapy* (HRT) in postmenopausal women, particularly with a combination of HRT using both estrogen and progesterone.[29] It is therefore reasonable to hypothesize that gender-affirming hormone therapy in trans women may increase their breast cancer risk. A large study conducted in the Netherlands reported that trans women developed breast cancer at a higher rate than cis men did but at a lower rate than cis women did. Conversely, trans men developed breast cancer at a lower rate than cis women.[30] Trans women who have taken or are taking gender-affirming hormones are encouraged to have screening mammograms every other year beginning at age fifty unless they have a family predisposition to breast cancer. The same is recommended for trans men who have not had a mastectomy (top surgery).[31] *Bottom line (and good news):* The absolute risk for breast cancer in trans people is low. *Bad news:* Trans people face some of the most glaring disparities when it comes to accessing health care, including cancer care.

People with physical and/or intellectual disabilities and neurodiverse people also face unique challenges when it comes to health care, including breast cancer care. A recent study reports that women with movement difficulties or complex-activity limitations had significantly higher rates of both breast and cervical cancer and had lower rates of recent mammograms and pap test screenings.[32] Patients with disabilities—including limitations in hearing, vision, cognition, and/or mobility—had lower rates of up-to-date mammography and cervical cancer screenings relative to patients with no disability, which may be related to mobility limitations or financial concerns for out-of-pocket costs.[33] Patients with autism spectrum disorder (ASD) face challenges related to health care and cancer screenings, including communication issues, particularly among individuals with nonverbal ASD, severe anxiety and associated behavioral challenges, and sensory-processing issues and sensitivities to screening procedures, and where the health-care provider lacks experience or understanding when it comes to dealing with ASD patients.[34]

I have personal experience with the challenges people on the spectrum face when it comes to receiving good health care. My son is on the spectrum, and routine visits to the pediatrician are anxiety-inducing and frightening for him, particularly because of his sensory-processing and -sensitivity issues. He's sensitive to loud noises and touch (shots are a challenge, and blood draws require calming medication and numbing cream), and like many people on the spectrum, anxiety and frustration often lead to meltdowns. Having providers who are familiar to him and with him (and familiar with autism in general) really helps.

In addition to the disparities in care that these populations face, the majority of breast cancer patients are female and therefore face pervasive sexism within the health-care system. No surprise, considering women face pervasive sexism in all aspects of life and in health care, from the ongoing battle for equal pay to the efforts to control or curtail women's reproductive health care. I experienced sexism when I was first diagnosed and asked my patient navigator about a comprehensive guide for new patients, envisioning something like a road map that delineates different treatment options for different diagnoses related to subtype, stage and grade, and preferences for reconstruction, including a time line for how long each step in the process may take. (How cool would that be?) According to my patient navigator, who balked at my suggestion, it was a terrible idea because it could, "scare or overwhelm patients with too much information."

Un-fucking-believable.

That attitude is so patronizing and infantilizing and smacks of "don't worry your pretty little head about such things." The insult was even worse because it came from another woman! *Newsflash:* Any woman who has received a cancer diagnosis is already terrified and confused.

Autism and Cancer

A fascinating link between ASD and mutations in oncogenes has been uncovered by investigators at the University of Iowa.[a] People with ASD actually have a higher rate of variation in DNA that encodes oncogenes, the products of which drive uncontrolled cancer cell growth. There's quite a large list of genes that have been identified to overlap between autism and cancer.[b] The really fascinating part is that while people with ASD have more variants in oncogenes, they have lower rates of cancer. In fact, researchers report that ASD is associated with a protective effect against cancer, particularly in boys and girls fourteen years of age or younger.[c] Understanding how this protection works could help us develop new treatments for cancer, as well as perhaps help us figure out how to use anticancer therapies targeting these genes to treat the more challenging symptoms of ASD.[d]

Sources

a. Benjamin W. Darbro et al., "Autism Linked to Increased Oncogene Mutations but Decreased Cancer Rate," *PLoS One* 11, no. 3 (March 2, 2016): e0149041, https://doi.org/10.1371/journal.pone.0149041, https://www.ncbi.nlm.nih.gov/pubmed/26934580; University of Iowa Health Care, "Study Discovers Link berween Cancer and Autism: Patients with Autism Have Increased Gene Mutations that Drive Cancer, but Lower Rates of Cancer," *ScienceDaily*, April 13, 2016, https://www.science-daily.com/releases/2016/04/160413120954.htm.

b. Jessica Wright, "Dozens of Autism Genes Have Cancer Connections," *Spectrum News*, June 10, 2016, https://www.spectrumnews.org/news/dozens-of-autism-genes-have-cancer-connections/; Jacqueline N. Crawley, Wolf-Dietrich Heyer, and Janine M. LaSalle, "Autism and Cancer Share Risk Genes, Pathways, and Drug Targets," *Trends in Genetics* 32, no. 3 (March 2016): 139–46, https://doi.org/10.1016/j.tig.2016.01.001, https://www.ncbi.nlm.nih.gov/pubmed/26830258.

c. Darbro et al., "Autism Linked."

d. Wright, "Dozens of Autism Genes"; Crawley, Heyer, and LaSalle, "Autism and Cancer."

What she needs—what every patient needs when faced with a health-care crisis—is information. Knowledge is power, and denying information based on sexist attitudes, arrogance on the part of health-care providers, or pure laziness or unwillingness to relay the information in a way that is accessible to the patient is grossly negligent, not to mention just plain gross. Another form of so-called benevolent sexism can be found in the misconception that anxiety over false positives is a *risk* associated with mammography screening; this belief can cause harm to women. "Preventing anxiety" has been cited by the United States Preventive Services Task Force (USPSTF) as justification for reducing routine mammography screenings among women between the ages of forty and forty-nine. Instead, we should be focusing on the very real, *scientifically validated* fact that breast cancer is a leading cause of premature death for women in their forties.[35]

Not surprisingly, "anxiety" isn't cited as a risk or factor used for routine prostate cancer–screening guidelines for men. (Hmm . . . I wonder what the difference could be . . .)

Talk about patronizing and infantilizing. Fortunately, other (female) investigators have debunked these biased screening criteria.[36] It's an uphill battle but one worth fighting. We patients are our own best advocates. If you feel your health-care team is being dismissive or not taking you seriously, withholding information you need to make good health-care decisions, remember: it's your body, and all decisions are ultimately in your control. And especially if your health-care team is not respecting your wishes or autonomy, *speak up.* Ask for a patient advocate. Let the health-care center know what's going on, and share your concerns. Consider switching care providers if possible. If not, see if your provider's center provides a patient navigator, or search for a breast cancer patient advocate who can help you.[37]

For some great information on how to be an effective advocate for your own health, check out *How to Be a Patient: The Essential Guide to Navigating the World of Modern Medicine,* written by registered nurse and public-health advocate Sana Goldberg.[38]

Speaking of autonomy, women who opt for aesthetic flat closure rather than conventional breast reconstruction (see chapter 4) can face unnecessary and infuriatingly sexist pushback or outright refusal to honor their surgical wishes. The heartbreaking and enraging stories range from women waking up from surgery with excess skin to horrific scarring due to lack of care for aesthetics because surgeons ignored patient wishes or thought they knew what was best.[39] This is not okay. As a patient, you know what is best for your body, and the decision is ultimately yours. Fortunately, advocates and survivors who have suffered at the hands of surgeons who refused to honor their wishes are working hard to raise awareness.[40]

And I'm doing my part by working with the breast cancer research and research-advocates programs at my institution to create a patient guide for new breast cancer patients!

I've devoted quite a few words to the ongoing cancer care disparities that exist for people of color, the poor, the uninsured, LGBTQIA+ folks, and disabled people. These disparities do not exist or operate in a vacuum, of course; they are part of larger social structures that afford default privilege to the White, the wealthy, the able-bodied, and the cis-heterosexual members of our society. Indeed, in their assessment of disparities related to the kinds and quality of health care received by minorities versus non-minorities, the *Institute of Medicine* (IOM) posits that "heath care disparities occur in the broader context of inequality."[41] In order to course correct and eliminate health-care disparities, we need to tackle the underlying systemic racism, bigotry, ableism, fear, and willful ignorance that obstruct change. We've made strides to be sure, but the facts and figures I've outlined above only scratch the surface of this problem of epic scale, and we have a long way yet to go.

What are the solutions?

In terms of the broader context of inequality, we need to keep the momentum of the antiracist movement, not to mention antihomophobia, antitransphobia and antiableist movements, moving forward in the United States and extend them to the sphere of health care. Diversity training and education for health-care providers needs to continue, and a diverse health-care workforce is necessary in order to improve outcomes and patient satisfaction.[42] Think it doesn't matter? Not only does cultural-competence training improve patient satisfaction, it also improves outcomes.[43] Moreover, efforts to increase the numbers of minority cancer researchers and cancer care providers to diversify the cancer workforce can help in a number of ways, including combatting implicit biases through diversity, which disproves false and unreliable biases and stereotypes, correcting the lack of cultural competence in research and cancer care, diversity- and inclusivity-fostered creativity and innovation, and reinforcement of similarities that transcend racial and ethnic lines.[44]

But what can *you* do personally? A great way to start is to lend your support to organizations that help communities of color, LGBTQIA+, and disabled breast cancer patients and survivors (I've provided descriptions and links at the end of this chapter). You can also vote for representatives who make eliminating disparities for these groups an active part of their platform, including and especially local and state representatives, to better help those folks in your community. Write your federal representatives to voice your support for universal healthcare coverage and for ending disparities in health care for marginalized and vulnerable populations. While you're at it, ask for more federal budget appropriations to the National Institutes of Health, which funds cancer research through the National Cancer Institute, and support increased funding for disparities research and interventions.[45] This is a double whammy in terms of support, since minorities in the field of cancer research are woefully underrepresented,[46] and many minority scientific investigators focus part of their research programs on eliminating disparities. So not only are you supporting minority patients, you're also supporting minority researchers and their valuable and important work.

Speaking of supporting minority researchers, the BlackinCancer organization is working to strengthen networks between Black people in cancer research and shining a light on Black excellence in cancer research and medicine.[47] Representation matters, and diversifying the cancer workforce is key to eliminating disparities in minority cancer-patient outcomes. In terms of supporting science-based public policy to overcome health disparities, the American Association for Cancer Research's 2020 *Cancer Disparities Progress Report* breaks down relevant federal agencies charged with tackling disparities in cancer care, as well as congressional caucuses actively engaged in reducing health disparities, including cancer, and policy initiatives that you can support through political activism.[48] Organizations like the American Association for Cancer Research and the American Cancer Society actively lobby for policies designed to reduce disparities as part of their mission, which is something you can support through donations.[49]

As I've already said, this chapter has only begun to touch on the depth and breadth of issues surrounding disparities in care. There are discrepancies within other racial and ethnic minority communities that I haven't covered, not to mention cultural barriers that lead to cancer disparities in the United States. My goals here are to (1) raise awareness, particularly among privileged White women who may lack experience or exposure to these types of disparities, (2) inspire empathy and self-directed research, because recognizing and acknowledging the problem is a critical first step to becoming part of the solution, (3) start a dialogue between patients and health-care providers about disparities they might be facing so providers can be part of the solution, and (4) empower all patients with information on how they can help tackle the problems of disparities in cancer care.

Organizations that Help Breast Cancer Patients and Survivors among Communities of Color, LGBTQIA+ Folks, and Disabled People

- *Sisters Network, Inc.*, brings awareness of the impact breast cancer has on the African American community and also provides a space for African American breast cancer patients to meet, bond, and receive support while receiving cancer treatment. http://www.sistersnetworkinc.org/.
- *The African American Healthcare Alliance* promotes awareness, early detection, and prevention while providing emotional and social support with culturally specific information and programs for women of color. https://www.aahafortwayne.org/.
- *Sisters by Choice* works to eliminate access barriers to screenings and quality care for breast cancer, including a mobile clinic to bring care to uninsured and underserved communities in Georgia. https://www.sistersbychoice.org/.
- *The Black Women's Health Imperative* is focused on improving the overall health and wellness of African American women and girls, providing outreach and curating Black women's health data

through its #WeRefuse initiative for breast cancer. https://bwhi
.org/.

- *2for2 Boobs, Inc.*, provides culturally relevant breast cancer information, resources, and educational materials for Black women;
the name is an acronym and call to action for self-examination, to
take 2 minutes 2 check your 2 (breasts). https://2for2boobs.org/.
- *Latinas Contra Cancer* works to create an inclusive health-care
system for cancer care in the underserved Hispanic and Latinx
population. http://latinascontracancer.org/.
- *The Latino Cancer Institute* promotes education, services, research,
and policies that impact Hispanics and Latinx people in the
United States when it comes to cancer. https://latinocancerinsti
tute.org/.
- *The American Indian Cancer Foundation* aims to eliminate the cancer burdens of Indigenous people by improving access to prevention, early detection, treatment, and support for survivors. https://
www.americanindiancancer.org/.
- *Asian American Cancer Support Network* provides education, support, and a diverse network of resources for Asian Americans
affected by cancer. http://aacsn.org/.
- *The American Association of People with Disabilities* is increasing
political and economic power for people with disabilities, supporting access to quality comprehensive and affordable health
care for people with disabilities as part of their mission. https://
www.aapd.com/.
- *The American Association on Intellectual and Developmental Disabilities* protects the universal human rights of people with intellectual
and developmental disabilities, supporting this group's access to
quality health care. https://www.aaidd.org/.
- *The National LGBT Cancer Network* educates, supports, and advocates for LGBT cancer patients and survivors and also maintains
a directory of LGBT-friendly cancer-treatment facilities. https://
cancer-network.org/.
- *The National LGBT Cancer Project* provides support and advocacy
for LGBT cancer survivors and supports equal and appropriate
access to cancer care for the LGBT community. https://www
.lgbtcancer.org/.

PART II

~

MY BREAST CANCER STORY

~

CHAPTER SEVEN

Nobody Expects the Spanish Inquisition, Or A Cancer Diagnosis

I've had my academic breast cancer researcher/professional lab rat[1] hat on for the first part of this book. It's my comfort zone. I can look at breast cancer cells in a dish under the microscope with professional detachment most of the time—though after my own diagnosis and after reading *The Immortal Life of Henrietta Lacks*, I can't help but wonder about the women behind these cell lines.[2] What were their lives like? What were their hopes, dreams, and aspirations? Do they—or did they—realize the impact their cancer tissues would have on the progress of science and the development of therapies to help future patients?

Patients like me.

In that spirit, it is time for me to share my own story.

It's time to get personal. I'm hanging up my researcher/lab rat hat to expose the ordinary, vulnerable woman beneath, whose own hopes, dreams, and aspirations were interrupted and threatened by breast cancer. I hope that, like the women whose cells I use in the laboratory to unlock the secrets of cancer, sharing my story can help future patients. Get ready for a long, convoluted journey through the US health-care system, navigating a series of stressful and often painful tests, information overload, and raging anxiety that emerged after I was told I had invasive breast cancer. Disaster is a sneaky beast that can strike on sunny days, on celebration days, and, in my case, on a random Thursday.

Believe me, when I was told I had cancer, it didn't matter that I'd spent twenty years already studying this disease. I was as shell-shocked, confused, numb, and terrified as any human receiving a cancer diagnosis. The only difference between me and the average lay patient, let's say, was that I proceeded to barrage my doctor with Science Questions. (More on that later.)

The answers I got didn't matter at the time. I couldn't hear or process the answers anyway. Hell, I couldn't even see my doctor or the files she held through a haze of tears. In spite of my background and knowledge base—which has been both a blessing and a curse—I was as scared and uncertain as any person who first hears the words, *You have cancer.*

The day I got my diagnosis—April 19, 2018—started out as a normal, hectic day. My only goal for the day was to get through it without being late for anything. (I was too busy to focus on dreams and aspirations.) As one of two working parents with full-time jobs in a household with two school-aged children (one with ASD/ADHD and the other knee-deep in rehearsals for a school play), I was and still am constantly on the move. That morning, my husband, Patrick, and I tag-teamed getting the kids ready for school. As usual, there were lots of repeated instructions (like *Find your backpacks and shoes like I asked you two ten minutes ago and like I ask you to every freaking day*), rushing to find my keys and phone (one of them disappears every day, without fail), and reminding my darling children that their father is *right there* and that he too can answer their questions, especially before mom's had her coffee. (I still have to remind them. I'm the go-to parent. It is my gift. It is my curse.)

In the middle of the chaos, Patrick and I chatted with excitement about the upcoming middle-school play while double-checking backpacks and binders and doing all the same mundane things we always do during our chaotic morning routine. We had too much to do. *I* had too much to do. Story of my adult life as a working mom and academic researcher—but somehow I would manage. I always did.

That day, I had to fit in a scheduled follow-up with my original breast surgeon—a long-haired, bubbly, and vivacious woman with kind eyes and a winning smile who defied all surgeon stereotypes. We had a great rapport and had already been through a lot together. Ever since I began having regular mammograms at the age of forty, I'd had issues. My breast tissue was dense, the internal landscape filled with strange little spots that looked like clusters of concentrated stars (see chapter 3, figure 3.1), galaxies in the universe of my body that were probably nothing to be concerned about, but the radiologist would review the data and let me know for sure.

Before I get into the nuts and bolts of D-Day—diagnosis day—I need to provide a little context, a brief history of my breast issues since I started getting regular mammograms.

As I mentioned in chapter 3, two of those spots found through routine screenings had turned out to be nothing, as is the most common outcome. By diagnosis day, I had already been through numerous screenings, breast-ultrasound exams, three ultrasound-guided biopsies, and a lumpectomy. That seems like a lot in retrospect, but it was my normal, and I had taken it all in stride. I was a breast cancer researcher, after all. This was practicing what I preached, and I used the same curiosity and hunger for new knowledge that drives me as a scientist to cope with the medical stuff in my life—stuff that I accepted as a necessary nuisance.

I always asked if I could see images from my exams—a request that my fantastic nurses and techs always honored. I got copies of my mammogram images on a CD along with copies of breast-ultrasound images. The ultrasound exams were similar to what I'd experienced each of the times I'd been pregnant, only instead of running the wand over my lower abdomen to look for a baby, the wand ran over my breast looking for abnormal structures (as detailed in chapter 3). While stretched out on a hospital bed, one boob or another exposed and covered with the cold, gooey gel they apply to the area being probed, I asked questions, craning my neck to see the screen until the kind radiologists and techs would move it and talk me through the process, what they were looking for, what we might be seeing on the screen. It was a great distraction, especially when the radiologist performing the biopsy inserted the needle into the suspicious lesion to extract a small portion for a pathologist to evaluate.

The local anesthetics always worked well, so I felt pressure without much pain, and I took advantage of my time under the ultrasound wand to learn about the clinical side of breast health. I knew about how breast cells grow in a dish and in a mouse, and I had seen benign lesions and cancers in tissue sections under the microscope. But seeing the internal workings of a human breast—my breast—was uncharted and fascinating territory. I had so many questions: *Is that a cyst? Why do they form? Oh, I see it—that area that looks like a little pocket of black emptiness in a sea of wavy, undulating lines on the screen that reminded me of the ocean. Yes, I see what you mean. The borders around the suspicious spot do look round and regular. Wow, you suctioned up a lot. I can't even see the spot anymore.*

That's good, right? Small is good?

My first suspicious lesion, detected after my first mammogram in 2014, at the age of forty, turned out to be a *fibroadenoma* in my right breast, a fairly common form of benign breast disease (BBD) that around 10 percent of women may have without even knowing it.[3] I'd had my first ultrasound-guided biopsy with this pesky little growth, which allowed my health-care team to identify it as a benign, fibrous growth that shouldn't give me any problems. These lesions aren't a sign that a woman will get breast cancer, so I wasn't worried. My health-care provider told me we'd just keep an eye on it, check it every year with my annual screenings to make sure it wasn't growing or changing shape. It got a little bigger over the next couple of years, but not enough to be worrisome. You can see what it looked like in 2016 in chapter 3, figure 3.3 (left panel).

My second lesion, detected in 2016 when I was forty-three years old, turned out to be an *intraductal papilloma*—a small, benign tumor that forms in a milk duct in the breast and is made of gland and fibrous tissue as well as blood vessels.[4] Before I knew the diagnosis and was waiting for biopsy results, I experienced a lot of stress and worry. My left breast had become sore and tender, and a worrisome discharge the color of pale blood leaked from the nipple. I called my breast surgeon and made an appointment for the following week, using Tylenol and work as a distraction by day and WebMD by night, ruminating over what this could be.

Yes, I was aware of the dangers of surfing this source of information and should've known better, but I'm human too. Was it cancer? I'd heard of Paget's disease of the nipple, a rare form of breast cancer with similar symptoms, but I also knew it could just as likely be a papilloma, so I waited (not so patiently) to find out whether I had a condition that was little more than a nuisance, a form of cancer, or something else entirely.

This was my first true scare. I had been through a lot with my breasts, from the time they had first developed, through their role in the joys and pleasures of sex, through nursing my two children; they'd never let me down. I could trust them. That trust wasn't exactly broken yet but cast into doubt. It's kind of like when you think your boyfriend might be cheating on you: intuition tells you something might be wrong, you've seen a few signs—distance, strange phone calls and text messages, followed by wild and out-of-character romantic gestures—but you don't have anything concrete, so you're stuck in limbo. My left breast may or may not have betrayed me, but I needed more evidence, and my surgeon was the private investigator who would follow it and examine, document, photograph, and build a case that would either clear it or indict it.

Fortunately, my breast was in the clear this time. I experienced my first surgery—a lumpectomy to remove the papilloma. Because the papilloma site was so close to my nipple, the surgeon was able to make an incision along the lower border of my *areola*, the darker skin surrounding the nipple, to hide the scar. Waking up from anesthesia, I felt fine. The pain was gone, replaced by a blissful numbness that left me on a pleasant cloud of contentment. I could rest. I would experience a different kind of soreness, but, as my '80s aerobics instructor would have said, it would be "a good hurt." Feel the burn, know that your body is repairing itself, that soon you'll be back to normal, like it never happened.

The nerve endings around my nipple had other ideas.

I noticed the changes in nipple sensation about a week after surgery while tending to the surgical site but assumed it was just residual pain from the incision. But as weeks went by and the responses to touch remained different, I began to realize that the changes might be long term or permanent. It didn't hurt, exactly, but it felt strange. The stroke of a finger or tongue sent electric shocks of bizarre sensation through my body along with the familiar, delicious pleasure. My surgeon told me it could take a year or more for full healing, and I assumed that included nerve endings. It wasn't the same, but it wasn't a deal breaker. I could, and would, work around it, as would my patient and loving husband. Over the next several months, I experienced phantom stabbing pains, more of those tiny electric-shock sensations, deep aches and soreness, and moments of intense relief followed by deep terror, like a near miss on the road (you swerve just in time to avoid the car barreling down the road toward you, pull over, heart pounding so hard you know it's going to burst from your ribcage, having narrowly avoided the unthinkable).

But eventually, I moved on. This was my new normal, and, all things considered, it was wonderful to have dodged the bullet that is cancer.

So, after a routine mammogram in 2018, I was neither surprised nor particularly scared when I was called back for more testing. I'd been down this road before and had become a bit of an amateur ultrasound enthusiast. The staff and I had established a great rapport at both radiology locations, and I often served as a training exercise for new technicians, chatting about work, kids, what on earth was up with Tennessee weather, how much I liked the tech's hair/nails/earrings—girl talk. The radiologist working with me that day was familiar, a woman who exuded calm competence that immediately put me at ease. She asked how I was doing, chatted with me about my plans for the week, and listened as the technician, who'd located the spot in question, showed her images captured on the small computer screen.

The spot looked familiar to my untrained eye—a dark, empty space in the ocean waves of my breast tissue, bobbing in and out of focus as the ultrasound wand rolled back and forth, pushed harder, then pulled back, allowing it to flicker in and out of focus (see chapter 3, figure 3.3, right panel). Blink, and you'd miss it. Then, the radiologist did something unexpected: she added more gel and casually moved the wand to the side of my left breast and around my armpit.

"That tickles." I apologized awkwardly as I'd wiggled and possibly squeaked in response. "What are you looking for?"

"Oh, just checking around," she reassured me.

I was a breast cancer researcher; I *knew* what was in that area. The lymph nodes that collected excess fluid from my left arm and breast were clustered there. One of the first places breast cancer spreads when it escapes the confines of normal tissue structural boundaries is to nearby lymph nodes. But I wasn't thinking about cancer at the time;

after all, this wasn't my first go-round. The technician and radiologist were calm, laughing and joking with me about my ticklish armpits and schoolgirl giggle. I also wasn't surprised or particularly concerned to learn that I would be having another ultrasound-guided biopsy—my fourth. My breasts were dense and prone to fibroadenomas, weird papillomas, and, thanks to a seatbelt injury from a car crash in 2017, something called *fat necrosis*, where injured squishy, bouncy fat cells had died after the trauma, resulting in internal scar tissue.

This was just how my body worked, and probably middle age was catching up with me.

I was forty-five, on the long march to menopause, entering a chapter of my life that I found strangely exciting and liberating. My children were growing, becoming more independent. They needed me, but not every moment, and they were spreading their wings and spending more time on their own, with friends, with their own activities that didn't involve me or Patrick. My career was going well—as was my progress toward tenure—I had recently lost twenty pounds and was on a health kick and feeling really good physically and mentally, and I had time to write (my side hustle is writing fiction; look me up under D. B. Sieders if you like reading urban fantasy and paranormal romance). I was looking ahead, always moving, and always moving forward. Little slowed me down in life.

Several weeks after the ultrasound screening, I had my fourth biopsy, performed by a new (to me) radiologist—a kind man with a gentle touch and great bedside manner. He was joined by a wonderful nurse wearing pink scrubs and a wide smile who put me at ease. I took my place on the table, watched the screen as the ultrasound wand found the pesky spot in question, marveled as I watched the needle that delivered anesthetic do its job and as the needle collected the biopsy, a small portion of the suspicious tissue that would then be sent to a pathologist to determine if it was benign or possibly malignant. As I watched the screen, my nurse took my hand in hers and squeezed each time the radiologist inserted the needle and moved it around.

I was a rational person, and, again, I didn't think this was a big deal. I'd been down this road before. But that human touch, such a simple gesture, made my eyes sting. I've carried the memory of this small kindness with me through my three-year adventure with breast cancer, along with the conversation with the radiologist about life: *What did I do for a living? Oh, you're a breast cancer researcher. Let me walk you through what I'm doing here. How many kids do you have? How old are they? What do they like?* I don't remember details, but I remember the easy flow of conversation, the cadence of his voice, and the soothing effect it had on me. I felt like a person—like I was a part of the team that would determine what was going on with my body. We were all in this together.

I don't know if my nurse that day offered the same comfort and gentle touch to all of her patients or if she suspected the results would show cancer. I suspect my radiologist knew, but I didn't go back to ask, and I'll never know for certain. In the end, it doesn't matter. What mattered at the time, and what matters in retrospect, is compassion.

I cannot stress enough how important it is for health-care professionals to remember that the person on the examination table is a person—a human being with aspirations, with people who love them, people who depend on them—and that it is just as important to engage with the human being as it is to tackle the disease or health challenge. This radiologist got it.

But not all do. Another radiologist I later worked with—the one who eventually confirmed the location of the cancer and its features before I consulted with my new breast surgeon—became flustered with me when, as a coping mechanism, I made a joke during her spiel about the exam that she was about to perform. She sighed, sounding annoyed, asked if I could just let her get through her explanation before I asked questions or made conversation. I was *floored.*

Here I was, sitting on yet *another* bed, preparing for another undignified examination that involved my lying half naked and covered in goo as I faced one of the most terrifying diagnoses in human experience, and she was scolding me for *interrupting her speech.* I'm sure it was the same speech she delivered to all patients, and I get it; it's important for doctors to tell patients exactly what they're about to do and why it's important and to make sure the patient understands and can explain what the doctor said in the patient's own words.

But . . . I've got to be honest—that was the first time in this process that I felt like a piece of meat.

My fear, my uncertainty, my terror about what the future might hold for me—none of it mattered to her, if the way she was treating me was any indication. To her, I was a number, just another case to get through in an overloaded system. The care she gave me was a far cry from the soothing voice and gentle touch I'd left behind when, for insurance purposes, I'd had to switch health-care providers.

I wasn't angry at her—at least, not at first—but in that moment, I shut down. She'd made it clear to me that questions were not welcome, that my attempts to cope and establish a rapport through humor were not appropriate, that I was throwing *her* off *her* rhythm. Later, when I had time to think on it, I wanted to go back and scream, "Mother-fucker, I have *cancer*! I get to talk, I get to question, I get to do whatever I need to do in order to deal with this because, after all, I'm the whole reason we're both here right now!"

Health-care providers, what she did? This is a great example of what not to do.

Now, backward on the time line, to D-Day. I was sitting on the exam table, cell phone in hand, scrolling through Facebook, annoyed that I was there. I was missing work—again—and had a tight schedule—as usual, with grant deadlines to meet, half-finished manuscripts to write, experiments to finish, data to analyze, and important Science Shit to do. I was irritated that I'd probably have another spot to keep an eye on—or, at the very worst, need another lumpectomy in my janky left boob. I'd already had that papilloma removed, and we were keeping an eye on a benign but possibly growing fibroadenoma in my right breast. I didn't have time for this. I needed to go home, get the house ready for my parents' visit (they were coming to town to see my daughter's play), pick up my son from school, figure out what we were all going to do for dinner, and prep for a very busy next day, when I would need to catch up with all the work I was missing. *Cancer* was the furthest thing from my mind.

My surgeon, who had performed my lumpectomy in 2016, walked into the room, and, for the first time, she didn't automatically ask how I was. Being a polite Southern gal, I naturally said, "Hi, how are you?" Her smile, which wasn't as bright as I'd expected, faltered, and she said, "I'm fine. I have your biopsy results back. You have cancer."

I stared at her, wondering if I'd misheard. I'd expected another fibro-adenoma—or some nuisance. Not *cancer*. This had to be a mistake. I was only forty-five. The greatest risk factor for most cancers, including breast cancer, is age.[5] Women sixty-five years old have a higher relative risk of developing breast cancer than women younger than sixty-five,[6] and I was twenty years younger than that. I didn't smoke or drink to excess, and while I was overweight (*read:* fat), that risk factor is greater in postmenopausal women. I was still getting regular periods, so no worries there. While I was older than thirty when I'd had my first child, I had breastfed both of my children for six to eight weeks, so I figured those cancelled each other out. (Not sure if that's true, but it was what I thought; very unscientific of me, I know.) Physical activity wasn't an issue, especially given my recent weight loss and health kick. I had no genetic history of breast cancer, but I'm taller than average, which is apparently associated with increased risk. And while I had mammo-graphically dense breasts and that pesky papilloma in my history, my docs had always assured me my risk was relatively low.

I wasn't supposed to have breast cancer.

This was supposed to be just another nuisance lesion I'd have to deal with, not some terrifying disease, the "big C," one of the three plagues of Western society, along with cardiovascular disease and metabolic disease (like diabetes).

She handed me a tissue. I hadn't even realized I was crying.

"I'm sorry—I didn't ask how you were when I first came in," she said, taking my hand. "It didn't make sense, since I had to deliver bad news."

I nodded. Then I went into full-on panic mode, which for me con-sisted of a barrage of rapid-fire questions.

"Is it DCIS or invasive? Is it ER/PR positive? HER2 negative? How big is it? How fast is it growing? Did they do Ki67 staining? How long has it been there? I mean, on average, breast tumors have to grow around five years before you can see them on a mammogram. I know that. This thing was here when I had the papilloma and lumpectomy to remove it last year, so how did we not see it?"

At this point, my surgeon put her hand on my shoulder and told me to breathe in through my nose; hold it for three counts—good, good—now out through your nose slowly. Again. Again. Good. We're going to go over all of this, I promise, but right now, just breathe.

I did, but all I kept thinking was, *How am I going to tell my kids I have cancer?*

After a few more deep breaths, we went over my pathology report. I had invasive ductal carcinoma, IDC, that was positive for both hormone receptors, estrogen receptor and progesterone receptor. It was strongly positive for Ki67, a marker of rapid growth, but since it was also so strongly positive for estrogen receptor, it would likely respond well to estrogen-blocking therapies. That was a good sign. We didn't know yet whether it was positive for HER2, a cell-surface receptor that induced rapid growth and made breast cancers more aggressive but also responded to targeted therapies. I was likely stage I, an early stage, which was good. We'd need more information, which we would get when we surgically removed the tumor.

We talked briefly about what I might want to do in terms of surgery (including the surgical options covered in chapter 4), and then she told me she was going to leave the room for a moment so I could call my husband. She would be back to check on me in about fifteen minutes, to see if I was okay to drive home or if I needed Patrick to come and get me. I closed down Facebook on my phone and scrolled through my favorites list to call Patrick.

"Hey," he said, his voice cheerful and pleasant as always. "All done? On your way home? What did they say?"

"Hey, babe. I'll be home soon," I said. Then, almost as an afterthought, I said, "And I have cancer. I'm okay. I think it's going to be okay. We caught it early, so it's probably going to be okay. Don't tell the kids yet. Ana needs to focus on her play, and Jason will freak out, which is unnecessary, because I'm going to be okay."

I stopped there since I didn't want him to hear my voice crack. I had a lump in my throat the size of a golf ball, and by now I was snot-crying. I had to be strong, though; I was a cancer researcher, a professional, and I understood more about this disease than most people. If I stayed strong and I pretended I wasn't worried, then he wouldn't worry. No one would worry. *It was all going to be okay.*

I had no idea if that was actually true, but it was the mantra going through my head and battling with the competing dark voice saying, "This is it. Put your head between your knees, and kiss your ass goodbye while the universe laughs at the irony."

Being an airline pilot, Patrick has been trained to be cool under pressure. It's in his nature to be the voice of reason—the rational, solid, competent presence in a crisis situation. He's talked me down from many ledges in our shared life, and right then I was filled with desperate hope that he could do that again—and simultaneously paralyzed by the fear that this time would be different. Would this be what broke us? Would it break *me*?

After a long pause, he said, "Okay . . . okay. I'm making myself captain of Team D Beats C. You okay to drive? I can come get you, but if you're okay to drive, come home. We've got this."

Not *You've* got this. *We've* got this. Those three powerful words made all the difference to me. They still do.

Soon, my surgeon came back into the exam room, and she also spoke with Patrick on the phone. And now I was ready to go home, see my daughter's play, visit with my parents, put aside this awful and somehow-not-yet-real news, and fall into the arms of my amazing husband. We were in this thing *together*.

Thank goodness for that, because I had no idea what I was in for.

CHAPTER EIGHT

~

New Boobs, New You?
The Toll Breast Cancer
Takes on Your Mental Health
and How to Deal with It

I covered the science and some practical considerations for cancer treatments specific to hormone receptor–positive breast cancer in chapter 5. It would be easy to leave it at that, and emotionally safer. Breast cancer hurt me, humbled me, and left me vulnerable, just like it does for every human being who battles this disease. Under the guise of being "rational," I spent the greater part of a year maintaining as much detachment from what was happening to me and my body as possible. I approached diagnostics, surgeries, and treatments as an intellectual pursuit, asking questions and learning all I could as a weird sort of hands-on research experience (where I was the freaking guinea pig) to augment my understanding of breast cancer in the context of my work.

It seemed like as good a way to cope as any.

Was it healthy? Insofar as it allowed me to get through the process with my sanity intact—that is to say, I'm as sane today as I ever was(n't)—it was healthier than denial, withdrawal from family and friends, or drowning my sorrows with wine (and rum and tequila and vodka). But I was straight-up in avoidance mode: I told myself I was okay. My prognosis was good, so I would be okay.

Sure, I'm a little nervous about surgery, I'd think, but I'll be okay. Yeah, maybe staying up until 2:00 A.M. three nights in a row working on my fiction writing side hustle wasn't the smartest idea, but it's what

111

you do as a writer. I'm totally okay. What if I have to have chemo? Well, we'll just have to wait for the Oncotype test results, so there's no use dwelling on it. I'm too busy to dwell on it anyway. I've got shit to do. I mean, I'm *always* busy. Always have been a doer, a mover and a shaker, a bitch on wheels.

Staying busy is good. It's productive. It means I don't have to think about the fact that I have cancer.

I have cancer.

Shit. I am *not* okay.

When that hit me—that I had cancer and was not okay—I realized that I needed help.

I'd had therapy before. Postpartum depression (PPD) had hit me hard after the births of my two children, and I had struggled with depression and anxiety for as long as I can remember, even before I had a name for the tangled web of conflicting emotions in my head. I had spiraled into a deeper depression with crushing anxiety when I'd entered graduate school. Oddly enough, I hadn't thought much of it at the time, since my circle of fellow graduate-student friends was chronically stressed-out as well. We were a bunch of overachievers, perfectionists, pathological workaholics who spent long days and late nights in our laboratories learning (often the hard way) how to do Science. We were all cucumbers with anxiety, and many of us—like me—managed it all with medication offered through the student health center. They offered counseling services too, but I hadn't been willing to open up to the older White male psychiatrist on staff who started all of our med management visits with, "How's your irritability?"

I assumed *irritability* was code for "You're being a difficult woman, so let's get you some meds for the sake of everyone around you."

I took the meds and silently wished the shrink to fuck off. Meds helped, but they were only one piece of the puzzle. I managed my anxiety and depression, but it became increasingly difficult to fight performance pressure and imposter syndrome during my postdoctoral training years, which coincided with the birth of my children.

It took thirty-three years before I finally went to therapy. My only regret in going to therapy was that I hadn't gone to therapy sooner.

What did I learn? For starters, I learned I wasn't alone. I became a mother before social media really took off, so I didn't have the benefit of the wonderful moms-supporting-moms Facebook groups. I was surprised to find that PPD was pretty common, as were anxiety and depression. Instead of being weak or harboring a dirty little secret, I actually shared a burden with many successful people, I learned, who are functional, fun, funny, charming, and smart, all while hiding their struggles. Some of us smile, laugh, and joke while our inner selves are curled up in a fetal position in a dark corner of our souls. Others eat or drink our feelings or self-medicate with drugs, compulsions, and too much work. Staying busy is my go-to (along with eating my feelings). If I'm busy, I'm not thinking. If I'm not thinking, my brain can't tell me lies that leave me crying in my closet on a random Thursday.

I went back to therapy just after my cancer diagnosis, though I (foolishly) stopped going after I found out I didn't need chemo. The therapist I was seeing at the time told me that cancer would push me up against a wall, get in my face, and ask, "What are you made of?" What was I made of? I didn't have an answer for her at the time, but the question stuck with me. I've spent the greater part of the past three years trying to come up with an honest answer. Scratch that—honest *answers* plural. The question is too big for just one answer.

What am I made of? If you'd asked me before cancer, I would have told you I was made of wine, coffee, and dirty jokes. In a more serious mood, I might have answered that I'm made of pathological persistence and a stubborn resolve to be the best I can be and to make a difference in the world. Before cancer, I'd never faced a challenge I couldn't out-think, outwork, outsmart, or simply walk away from.

But I couldn't walk away from this. Cancer didn't care how smart I was or how driven. Those clusters of tumor cells growing inside of me only cared about their own survival. Cancer didn't care about my kids, who put on brave faces but were scared about losing their mother. Cancer didn't care about my husband, who was strong for my sake but still worried about the uncertainties that come with this awful disease. Cancer didn't care about my hopes, dreams, and aspirations.

I couldn't outwit cancer, and I couldn't appeal to cancer's better nature; it doesn't *have* a better nature. Cancer was a part of me that had broken ranks and gone rogue, relentlessly growing and invading the healthy parts of my body that were still a part of the collective they had once served. And in my fight against cancer, it was sure to take more than a few pieces of me with it.

That became my first answer to the big question. What was I made of? I knew I was no longer made of *me*. Shortly before surgery, I realized that my body was no longer my own. Even with a lumpectomy (the first time around), the breasts I'd woken up with were not mine. As soon as my surgeons had marked my skin, I'd relinquished ownership of my breasts, along with the image of myself I'd always carried (see chapter 16, figure 16.3). True, I hadn't always loved my body or had the best relationship with it, but it had always been *mine*. We'd grown together, gone through the adventures of youth, the joys of dating and marriage, borne two children, and reached middle age together. I had accepted my wrinkles, muffin top, and sagging breasts as a continuation of the journey, certain that we'd march toward old age with mutual respect and trust.

But after cancer surgery and radiation, while I could look at my body objectively and appreciate the pleasing shape of my new breasts beyond the scars, they still weren't "mine" (see chapter 16, figure 16.4). This wasn't "me." Phantom pains and the sting of healing nerves only added to the alien feeling of not belonging in my own skin. By the time I was diagnosed with residual disease almost two years later, I had almost moved past the separation I'd been feeling with my body, only to experience it all over again, and with even greater intensity as I lost my left breast entirely. My surgeons were kind and incredibly skilled and are still working diligently to give me back some semblance of what I'd lost, but I had to come to terms with the fact that part of me was forever lost, and I had to grieve before I could accept my body and myself as it was and as it continues to change.

That acceptance is still a work in progress.

As of this writing, I have had five surgeries, including the most recent revision procedure after autologous reconstruction. The grafted tissue from my thigh gave me a new breast, but it wasn't smooth, and it wasn't the same size as the right breast in spite of a lift (see chapter 16, figure 16.6). The first revision to correct this involved liposuction and fat grafts to plump up the new left breast, followed by another lift on the right side—the third time that breast has been lifted (see chapter 16, figure 16.7). It's much better, but we're still not done. I look at my bruised and battered body, and though the shape and contours defy the reality of my age, I mourn for my old self and wonder how much more my body can take.

So, what was I made of?

Some days, I was made of scars that crisscrossed what was left of my breasts and extended to my armpits. During and after radiation, I was made of fatigue and of skin that went from red and raw to tight and tough as unoiled leather. Gone was the soft supple texture. Would my husband be okay touching it? I wasn't okay with how it looked or the loss of sensation, which fed into the vicious cycle of damage to my body image.

What was I made of?

After I entered medically induced menopause with Lupron and AIs, I was made of fire and sweat and tears. Lupron is a gonadotropin-releasing hormone analogue, or GnRH, which means it mimics gonadotropin-releasing hormone; it blocks release of gonadotropin by the hypothalamus. Gonadotropin tells the pituitary gland to make luteinizing hormone (LH) and follicle-stimulating hormone (FSH), which in turn signals to ovaries or testes to make estrogen and progesterone in biological females or testosterone in biological males. No GnRH, no sex hormones. Lupron stopped my body from making estrogen, and AIs stopped other tissues in my body like adrenal glands, fat, breast tissue, and muscle from making estrogen.

Stopping estrogen production in my body, among other things, makes me really fucking hot.

A volcano erupted from deep within the core of my body and radiated out in waves that left me panting and shaking. "Hot flashes" or "hot flushes" are bullshit names for the process by which the loss of estrogen somehow convinces the hypothalamus—aka the body's thermostat—that the body is too hot. When your body thinks it's too hot, your heart rate increases, the blood vessels close to the surface of your skin dilate to circulate more blood in an effort to get rid of heat, and your sweat glands ramp up to cool you off. But you don't really need to cool off, and in the aftermath of a hot flash you're left soaking wet and miserable. Even worse, you get *cold* after hot flashes. Sometimes I'm made of multiple layers of clothing and wardrobe changes.

Menopausal women can use hormone-replacement therapy, HRT, to alleviate the symptoms of menopause like hot flashes, as well as insomnia, loss of bone density, appetite changes, and high blood sugar. Because being hot isn't bad enough, right? Let's lose sleep, get brittle bones, *and* get diabetes! However, women like me, with hormone receptor–positive breast cancer, can't use HRT because it could make any leftover cancer cells hiding in our bodies grow. Sometimes, I'm made of bitterness and jealousy because there's no relief for the hell of medically induced menopause.

What was I made of? Before cancer, it was warm hugs, belly laughs, and a lust for life and all the experiences it has to offer. But breast surgery puts warm hugs on hold during the healing process, as does radiation. Side hugs aren't the same, and hugs from the back just don't quite have the same all-encompassing warmth as a from-the-front, soft, breast-cushioned hug. I'd gotten those hugs back after the first two surgeries (lumpectomy for benign papilloma and lumpectomy for cancer), but I had to give them up again after mastectomy, autologous reconstruction, and the first round of revision surgeries.

I miss them. I hope I get them back soon. I think I will.

As for belly laughs, I'm grateful for my family, friends, an amazing circle of survivor sisters and brothers, and my own sick sense of humor. After watching Tig Notaro and Wanda Sykes, two incredible comedians who had the guts to talk about their breast cancer experiences on stage, I started to laugh again.

Lust for life and experiences? That's a bit more . . . complicated. Cancer has an annoying way of putting your life on hold. Planning around surgeries, treatments, and medication side effects—like fatigue and crippling bone, joint, and muscle pain—sucks. Some days, I was the Energizer Bunny, ready to hike four miles and splash in a sun-kissed swimming pool later that evening. Other days I could barely uncurl my claw fingers that hurt like arthritis on steroids, let alone get out of bed to go enjoy a beautiful Saturday with my kids.

What was I made of? I was *every* woman, Wonder Woman, Super-woman—I'd just left my cape at the cleaners. I had long prided myself on being able to do it all and do it well. I could work a full day in the lab—a noble calling buried beneath reams of paperwork, endless meetings, and the never-ending quest for funding—and still come home to make a healthy meal, engage with my children, help with homework and chores, and be an amazing wife. Not that my husband was ever "that guy," the kind who's all too happy to sit back and relax while exploiting his wife's unpaid physical and emotional labor while patting himself on the back for sometimes doing the dishes. No, this being-Superwoman thing was all me. You see, I had something to prove. I'd grown up in the seventies and eighties, a time when women's liberation was telling us that we could do it all and be it all if only we worked hard enough. That philosophy morphed into '90s girl power and, later in the new millennium, told us to lean in. I embraced and reveled in all of it. Pushback from conservatives, misogynists, and doubters didn't daunt me; they fucking *motivated* me.

So being forced to slow down for breast cancer *did not compute*. The seismic disruption to the life I'd built for myself derailed my sense of self so deeply and profoundly that I'm still coming to terms with the aftermath. Being diagnosed with residual disease in February of 2020—the beginning of the COVID-19 era—has not helped. The world stopped moving. I stopped moving. I didn't deal well with that.

So, I went back to see a therapist, and with a lot of work fighting cognitive distortions like catastrophizing (assuming the worst outcome), control fallacy (believing I'm solely responsible for and in control of myself and my surroundings), and polarized thinking (believing it's all or nothing), I found out I was still made of determination, resilience, and hope. Other things that helped me through the dual crises of COVID and cancer were yoga and mindfulness meditation, narrowing my world to focus on my health and well-being and my family, and writing.

What am I made of? I'm made of persistence. Cancer hasn't stopped me in my tracks; it's just put me on pause for a while—and not even on a full pause. It's given me a new lease on life—as often happens when people face their own mortality—a new mission to fight breast cancer outside of the laboratory through advocacy and inside the laboratory with a renewed sense of urgency and focus on novel treatments that can feasibly be translated to the clinic.

I'm *still* made of coffee, wine, and dirty jokes—and thank goodness for that. Humor is a great coping mechanism that I highly recommend. If you can laugh in the face of cancer, then cancer can never truly defeat you. In that spirit, later on, in chapter 9, I'll share some of the funnier moments from my breast cancer journey and about my breasts.

But first, I'd like to dig deeper into what it means to cultivate wellness when you're faced with cancer.

Taking Care of Mental, Emotional, and Spiritual Health When You Have Breast Cancer

Finding out you have cancer is traumatic. It messes with your head and your heart as much as it messes with your body. After receiving my breast cancer diagnosis, I went through a phase of numbness, unable to access my feelings but painfully aware of the tightness in my chest and knots in my stomach. Those physical symptoms were a sign of what was to come—fear, anger, guilt, sadness, and grief. Fear was the first and most understandable emotion washing over me. There's nothing like being told you have a deadly disease to teach you fear. Like many cancer patients, I raged at the universe about the unfairness of my situation. After all, I'd maintained a fairly healthy lifestyle. I ate my fruits and veggies, minimized junk food, exercised semiregularly, didn't smoke, didn't drink excessively, and, aside from fighting a genetic predisposition to high blood pressure, I was doing well for my age. So why did *I* get cancer? What had I done wrong?

Guilt told me I had done plenty wrong, and reading list after list of risk factors for breast cancer didn't help. I was overweight. I'd given birth to my children after thirty. I'd only breast fed my children for six to eight weeks due to issues with cracked nipples, an infection, and low milk production—so, clearly, I'd stupidly skipped out on that measure of protection. Since I'd chosen a high-stress life, balancing work and career, I had brought this all on myself. And *because* it was my fault, my family was going to suffer. I knew that during treatment there were going to be long stretches of time that I wouldn't be able to take care of myself, let alone anyone else, which played upon one of my greatest fears—loss of independence and being a burden. How would the stress and worry affect my children psychologically? My son, who is on the autism spectrum and has ADHD, required a great deal of care and attention in order to thrive. My husband and I had managed the juggle through creative scheduling and teamwork.

Now, he'd have to take care of it on his own—or worse, my daughter would unfairly be asked to step up and step in.

If my prognosis changed based on what pathology found after surgery, would my life be cut short? Guilt at the prospect of leaving my children motherless, of missing milestones like graduations, weddings, the births of future grandchildren, of not being able to guide them through the transition from childhood to adulthood threatened to swallow me whole and send me spiraling into the abyss of despair. Sadness and grief over what I'd lost, what I might lose, and how it would affect the people I loved threatened the foundation of the tough, resilient, I-can-do-anything persona I'd constructed for myself.

Uncertainty was *not* my friend.

But how could I cope? How can *anyone* cope with the terror and unpredictability of cancer? There's no one right answer, no one-size-fits-all solution.

Many cancer patients and survivors find support and comfort from the larger community of survivors. Sharing experiences, having someone to email, call, message, or text who understands what you're going through can really help. Many cancer centers offer hotlines and helplines that can connect you to other survivors. Ask your health-care team about these resources. Organizations like Gilda's Club are great places to find community support as well as other practical resources to help during cancer treatments and recovery.[1] Check for a location in your area. They'll help you remember that you're not alone.

Others find support during cancer treatment from their faith communities, which in addition to offering prayers can offer support in the form of visits, preparing and delivering meals, and help with day-to-day activities to support the cancer patient and their family. Reach out to your faith leader for help and support; it's a vital part of their job, and they'll most likely be glad to help and organize support.

As for me, I found that a combination of therapy and mindfulness practice in the form of yoga was the solution. Using cognitive behavioral therapy (CBT)[2] to challenge cognitive distortions that I clung to in the face of fear, anger, guilt, sadness, and grief has been a lifeline. It was fine to be afraid; fear is a normal emotion and reasonable to experience in the face of a breast cancer diagnosis. But spiraling into predictions of worst-case scenario outcomes—or catastrophizing—isn't reasonable or healthy. With the help of my therapist, I was able to challenge these distortions with facts about my diagnosis, likely outcomes, and alternatives to the worst case. Anger is a normal emotion, but succumbing to bitterness at the unfairness of being diagnosed with cancer isn't healthy or productive. Neither was indulging in guilt and self-blame. As human beings, we look for patterns, reasons, and explanations for what happens in our lives, and we often cling to the illusion that we're somehow in control of them. At the end of his Netflix special, *Annihilation*, Patton Oswalt, another of my favorite comedians, shares the motto his late wife, author Michelle Eileen McNamara, lived by: "It's chaos. Be kind."[3] This philosophy helped see him through the incredibly painful loss of his wife, and he shared it with the wider world. What does it mean? That there's no rhyme or reason for what happens to us, be it the loss of a loved one, a catastrophic event, or a cancer diagnosis. We aren't in control. The best we can do in the midst of the chaos is to be kind. Spread kindness in your community, at work, at home, to random strangers in the grocery store, and, perhaps most importantly, to yourself. Instead of looking for reasons why you or someone you love got cancer, focus on what you can do to take care of yourself. For me, that kindness extends to helping others through advocacy work and through this book as well as in the laboratory. Never underestimate the healing power of kindness.

Sadness and grief are also natural emotions and normal reactions to a cancer diagnosis—emotions that I would argue need to be processed and endured. You cannot accept yourself postcancer until you mourn the loss or change of the person you were before cancer. It's okay to grieve over the loss of your body as it was, as well as to grieve over the lasting impact cancer has on your health and your outlook on life. The key is to then accept yourself postcancer and move forward. I'm not saying, "Just get over it already." (That kind of "advice" triggers a special kind of rage in me; more on that in chapter 15.) What I mean is that you should not let grief and sadness trap you. Sure, you may *never* be done grieving—just as we never really stop grieving for lost loved ones. The anguish will sneak up on you from time to time and try to suck you into a perpetual state of despair. Don't let it. Instead, try to focus on the amazing person you are; because anyone who battles cancer *is* amazing. No matter what it has taken from you, cancer hasn't defeated you. *You're still here.* Make the most of your time on this planet, and live to the fullest in whatever way is meaningful for you.

One really effective way to fight cognitive distortions and avoid being overwhelmed by negative emotions is mindfulness—which means being fully present in the moment without becoming overwhelmed by what's going on around us or within our own headspaces. Studies on the benefits of mindfulness and meditation show that it can help manage stress, anxiety, fatigue, mood, and sleep quality when combined with standard-of-care medical interventions.[4] I'm no good at conventional meditation, by which I mean sitting still and focusing on my breath without letting my thoughts wander. I've never been able to shut off my mind by just sitting and consciously breathing. But put me in a yoga pose that I have to focus on to maintain (i.e., not fall on my ass)? I can focus on my breath and be present in the moment all day!

No matter which of these interventions you choose—or something else entirely—don't forget to focus on your mental and emotional health. And be kind to yourself.

CHAPTER NINE

~

I Laugh in the Face of Cancer

A Few Funny Stories

As you may have guessed, in addition to keeping busy, humor is my go-to when it comes to coping with cancer and other adversities in my life. I recommend it. I don't take myself or anything else too seriously, as you'll see through some of my favorite funny, (hopefully) entertaining, often-cringeworthy, but always interesting (at least to me) stories. The lessons I took from these experiences were as follows: you've got to have friends, preferably ones as weird as you are; you should enjoy the beauty around you, especially when it comes in the form of a gorgeous health-care provider; and you should cherish the embarrassing, awkward, uncomfortable moments that let you laugh at yourself, with everyone around you, and in the face of trauma.

Laughter may not be the *only* medicine for a cancer diagnosis, but it's one of the best.

Booby Radar

As we covered in chapter 4, one of the more recent advances in breast surgery as of 2018 is the use of radar technology to help surgeons locate small tumors in a sea of healthy breast tissue. In the past, patients had wires jammed into their breasts on the day of surgery as a sort of fucked-up "X" marks the spot. Aside from being just plain horrifying, the wires implanted in the breast tissue could shift position, leading to missing diseased tissue and the need for re-excision. Today patients have the option of getting small reflector devices inserted into their breast tissue prior to surgery. I had three implanted into my body prior to surgery: two to mark tumor tissue in my left breast and one to mark a benign (but growing) fibroadenoma in my right. Since I was a candidate for oncoplastic breast-conserving surgery, my surgeon decided to go ahead and remove the fibroadenoma on the right since the plastic surgeon would have to work on the right breast for matching cosmesis. That was fine.

Or so I thought, until I found myself trapped in a chair while being stabbed repeatedly in the boob.

Okay, that sounds bad. My radiologists were and are consummate professionals, and I'm sure there's some medical-coding-worthy name for the procedure I endured, but what it *boiled down to* was being stabbed in the boob with ginormous needles, repeatedly.

Here's what happened.

It started out okay. They were able to implant one device near the fibroadenoma in my right breast, using ultrasound as a guide. Reclining on the gurney with my right arm elevated, I kept my eyes on the screen and watched along with the nurse and the radiologist as he first guided a needle full of lidocaine deep inside my breast tissue along a path that led to the lesion. Then I watched as he implanted the first SAVI device.[1]

As it had with the second tumor biopsy on my left breast, implanting the SAVI devices near the lesions proved a bit more complicated.

I entered the room wearing my robe and, thankfully, pants. The two people there, a kind radiologist and an even kinder nurse, tried to put me at ease. It worked at first. The room was dimly lit with soothing, soft illumination, which muted the harsh lines of medical equipment and generic walls, tiles, and cabinets. The hum of equipment sapping energy from their outlets also soothed, as did the recliner.

Even the mammography machine—a miniature version of the monstrosity of rotating plastic, metal, and intimidating large plastic plates of boob-flattening horror—seemed mundane. Of course, looks can be deceiving, as my first experience of mammogram-guided biopsy proved.

Side-story time. (Don't worry; it's also funny.)

As I said back in chapter 3, mammogram-guided biopsy (also called a *stereotactic* biopsy) combines a mini-mammogram with a needle-core biopsy: You basically put your boob through a hole in a modified gurney/hospital bed, which is then raised so the radiologist and nurse can work beneath you—like a car getting some shit done to the undercarriage. You are required to lie perfectly still and hold your breath multiple times for each image. There's a lot of noise—like if R2D2 were in the room with a sewing machine and some weird alien that feeds by suction. It sounded a little something like

Beep beep . . . boop . . . beep . . . beep . . .

followed by the sewing-machine sound, which I assumed was the needle moving around, based on the weird pressure and vague ache in the boob:

Chchchchchchchch . . . beep . . . [uncomfortable silence] *. . . chchchchch-chchch . . .*

Then came the most disturbing sound:

Schlllluuuuuurp.

There went tiny chunks of my boobies. (Ew.)

That last part is quite different from the "clicker," the collection mechanism used in the ultrasound-guided biopsy to collect core samples. The clicker makes a loud *clack* that the radiologist will warn you about so you don't jump off the table and cause massive injury to your needle-invaded breasticle. Stereotactic procedures are much quieter—aside from the whole *beep . . . boop . . . chchchchchchchch . . . schlllluuuuuurp* thing.

Back to the main story.

Like the biopsy, implantation of SAVI devices into my left breast had to be a mammogram-guided procedure. Unlike the mammogram-guided biopsy, this time I wasn't lying facedown on an elevated gurney with my left breast hanging down for easy access. Instead, I was asked to sit upright in a transformer-style medical chair with a pillow at my back, left breast in compression after several attempts to align the breast such that the radiologist could insert both needles and implant the devices in the same field.

I watched in horror and strange fascination as the radiologist jammed two mini-screwdriver-sized needles into my breast.

I'm talking waaaaaay the hell deep inside my breast. *While I watched.*[2]

Even better, while all of this is going on, the doc calmly asked me, "Do you feel pressure on the other side?" The *other side*, meaning he'd jammed the needle *all the way through my boob.*

Yeah. The big-ass needle had gone in one side and right out the other.

I answered yes—numb with shock at the horror-movie sight below me. Now, it's important to understand that all this time I felt nothing but vague pressure and a slight pinprick where the needles hit the other side of my boob; the lidocaine was doing its job. Also, these particular needles were smaller in terms of bore size than the biopsy devices had been. Still, looking at metal objects jammed into my breast tissue while I was immobilized and rather uncomfortable was pretty surreal. There wasn't a lot of blood, but, really, it only takes a little blood to induce a major freakout.

Fortunately, I had a job to do: We took approximately twenty to thirty images, and for most of these my mission—in addition to holding my breath when told—was to hold my right boob out of the line of the imaging beam. So, *to recap:* sitting upright, up close and personal to the mammography machine, with my left hand at my side and my right holding my right boob out of the way, leaning slightly into the machine lest I accidentally and/or in a delayed panic reaction yank my boob out of compression with the added horror of getting the two needles caught in the mammography apparatus and possibly tearing my breast out.

The nurse and doc noted how remarkably calm I seemed—and surprisingly, I was. It was that numb kind of frozen calm you get when you know bad stuff is happening that you can't stop so your brain shuts itself down until it's safe to process. Not that I was able to stop staring at the boob needles, but I was able to sit still, engage in conversations designed to distract me while the radiologist adjusted the positions of the needles between imaging sessions, and even laugh a little. They called me a trooper and said I was a great patient, and after patching me up with gauze and tape, I dressed, gathered my belongings, and drove a short distance to the Hollywood 27 Cinema to see *Deadpool 2.*

This was fitting, since (*spoiler alert!*), Wade Wilson—aka Dead-pool—entered the Weapon X program in order to cure terminal cancer. Not that mine is/was terminal, but I felt a sort of kinship with "the Merc with a mouth." I enjoyed popcorn and a ginormous soda (that had me running to pee near the end of the movie), but I still got back in time to see Deadpool regenerating the lower half of his body while negotiating with his erstwhile nemesis, Cable.

It was only when I returned to the car and began driving home that it hit me: adrenaline flooded my system, as my heart began racing. I pulled over, ran shaking hands over my body, including the pincushions formerly known as my breasts, and began laughing hysterically at the absolute absurdity of the situation. I called my husband, who told me I should probably come home, because we still needed to pack for our vacation. Though he *tried* to be understanding, what I needed in that moment was someone who *did* understand. I needed a survivor sister with a warped view of the world and a sense of humor as fucked up as mine. I needed Pam.

Pam Jasper was and still is my rock. She'd been through breast cancer before me and was my go-to for answers, support, a laugh, a stiff drink, and advice. She's my sister-by-choice and gal pal whose company always makes my day better. Sitting in the parking lot of the tackiest movie theater in Nashville, in the middle of what was most likely a panic attack, I needed Pam to talk me off this ledge.

PAM: Hey, girl! How'd it go?

ME: Great, but, um, I think I may be having a delayed freak-out? I was okay when I had the Cyborg Device put in on the right boob, but the needle going in one side of my left breast and out the other may have been too much.

PAM: *Long pause* Wait. What the hell did they put in you?

ME: Radar devices—like, these tiny little transmitter doohickies that are supposed to tell the surgeon where to cut. At least, that's what they told me. It's kind of a blur now. Wait, is it normal to close your eyes and see booby needles? This is definitely nightmare material.

PAM: Oh, my god, they microchipped you.

ME: Holy shit. What if they did? Like, do you think they're tracking me now?

PAM: *Glasses clinking in the background[3]* Dunno. Did you try calling the mother ship?

ME: Well, I would, but they didn't tell me how to activate the damned things. Should I just talk *into* my boobs? Do I need to squeeze them first? This should really come with an instruction manual.

PAM: *Excitement pours through the phone* Wait a minute. You said those things were Cyborg Devices. We may have this all wrong. I think they're turning you into the Terminator. But instead of Sarah Connor, you're on a mission to destroy *breast cancer*.

ME: You think so? The Terminator is pretty badass.

PAM: So are you. You're going to focus on those little Cyborg Devices, and you're going to tell those tumors that they're in your sights, you're locked and loaded, and you're going to terminate them.

ME: *Wiping my eyes and blowing my nose* Yeah. You're right. Fuck those tumors. I *am* going to terminate them.

PAM: Damn right you are. Now, are you okay to drive?

ME: Probably. You got a glass of wine waiting for me?

PAM: Glass of wine, gin and tonic, rum and Coke—I've got it all. Now get your Cyborg Boobs over here.[4]

That's how I managed to get through all of this.

Also, Ryan Reynolds is *amazing* in *Deadpool* and *Deadpool 2*. He's funny, charming, wildly raunchy and inappropriate (no wonder I love him), and just flat-out fun. He's also an incredible human being. He's raised some serious cash for cancer charities and research through contests for fundraising company Omaze and merchandise to support the Fuck Cancer Foundation. I wore my Fuck Cancer T-shirt the day of my first surgery and felt as badass as the Merc with a mouth. Thank you, Ryan Reynolds.

Inappropriate Flirting: The Socially Awkward Edition

I am not smooth. I am not sophisticated or socially adept. I can wear professionalism and normalcy for about an hour, but it's a thin disguise for my inherent and often-disturbing weirdness.

Reader, I can hear your screams of "Duh!" and "No shit." That is fair. If you've made it this far into the book, news of my tendency toward inappropriateness isn't some big reveal.

And my surgical experiences were no exception.

Prior to surgery, I needed to be injected with a tracer that would be absorbed by nearby lymph nodes, thus marking them for the surgeon so she could remove a few and send them to pathology to screen for cancer. Lymph nodes are the first location where breast cancer invades and spreads, so *sentinel-node biopsies* are essential for proper diagnosis of stage (as discussed in chapter 3). Preparation for the biopsy by injection of the tracers should have been no big deal—boring even. It is for most patients.

But not me.

Picture this: I'm decked out in my super-sexy surgical suit, complete with a hair cap and bright-yellow nonslip one-size-fits-all socks, and I'm not wearing makeup on my forty-five-year-old face. It's early, so my eyes are bleary, bloodshot, and probably crusty. (Yeah, I was totally at my best.)

I wasn't wearing underwear, either. #Smexy.

They wheeled me out of the prep room and through the waiting room, where I got to wave at my husband as they transported me to Nuclear Medicine, which is located in the coldest freaking corridor of the hospital. I work at the medical center, so I know. They parked me there, outside of the door in the freezing corridor, draped in a flimsy sheet, where I waited. The two corridors that intersect this one are pretty high traffic, so I got to smile and wave awkwardly at passers-by, hoping that the next person who came along wouldn't be someone I knew—like students or my boss. (The people I work with and teach are totally awesome and sympathetic, but the only thing weirder would be seeing one of my former med students coming in to perform or observe my *gyno* exam.)

Wishing I had my cell phone, I fidgeted, adjusted my sheet into something vaguely toga-shaped for my own entertainment, and waited.

And waited.

And waited.

Then the door opened, and out popped the head and torso of a tall, muscled, *gorgeous* man. Light hair somewhere between auburn and honey-colored, brilliant blue eyes, a bit of stubble on the chiseled jawline, and scrubs that fit in all the right places—he was a vision. It was totally wrong to stare, to objectify my health-care provider, and I couldn't blame drugs (I hadn't had any yet). Maybe it was stress. Or perhaps it was my mind latching onto something that would distract me from the prospect of getting a boob job I'd never asked for and hoping the cancer hadn't spread. I'd told hubby that if they found cancer in my nodes, they should shift gears and take the left breast off entirely by mastectomy.

I wouldn't know until I woke up, and that was a rather terrifying prospect.

So, through that lens, I ogled the beautiful man who'd been charged with injecting a radioactive tracer into the nipple of my poor, cancer-ridden left breast. He was as sweet was he was gorgeous, putting me at ease immediately with kind words delivered in a deep, rumbling voice. He wheeled my chariot wheelchair into the brightly lit room, which was slightly warmer than the hallway outside, and talked me through the procedure. I didn't pay much attention, to be honest; and neither did I pay a great deal of attention to the bulky equipment in the room, aside from a small table, above which some kind of diagnostic contraption hung.

"Are you ready?" Dreamboat asked, smiling.

"I'm sorry, what?" My cheeks heated. Fuck. Now he'd know I was admiring his physique and voice rather than listening to whatever instructions he'd apparently just given me.

He grinned, bright teeth gleaming in the harsh light of the room. There was just such a wonderful aura surrounding the man—not like a *literal* aura, because (a) auras don't exist and (b) I hadn't had any drugs that would produce an aura hallucination, but he carried with him an air of kind competence. And patience. (Good thing.)

"Let's get you on the table and get you comfortable, okay?"

Yes, my Medical Dreamboat . . . "Okay!" I actually said, and *giggled*, tucking a bit of hair behind my ear.

It might have been cute if my curly mop hadn't been shoved into an ugly hospital shower-cap thing. Lucky for me, he either didn't see my ridiculously not-smooth move, or else he was polite enough to just ignore it. He offered his muscle-bound arm and guided me out of the wheelchair—*Like a goddamned gentleman.*—and helped me settle my ass onto the table with the weird doohickey hanging over it.

The gown kept my bare ass covered and prevented it from coming in contact with the table, which was nice. But it was kind of like wearing an ill-fitting prom dress, which made it tough to stay balanced and move gracefully midrecline. Still, the moment was magical as Dreamboat settled me in and then turned to check his supplies. Being unbalanced (physically[5]), I slowly let my upper body fall while stretching my legs—perhaps showing a bit of calf as my gown rode up.

Then, all of a sudden, *boom.*

The back of my head slammed into the damned thing suspended above the table. It was hard enough to ring my bell. I saw stars. Then I saw Dreamboat's face close to mine, brows furrowed in concern and chiseled jaw clenched tight. He was worried.

I was mortified.

"I'm okay!" I said, my voice about two octaves higher than normal. "I'm such a klutz."

He nodded but then pulled me back up and stared into my eyes. I stared back, wondering if this was just a really weird anesthesia dream.

No such luck. Dreamboat pulled out a penlight, and it suddenly dawned on me that he was worried that I'd given myself a concussion. (Shit. This would go into his notes, which would then go into my medical record, and all of my health-care providers would think I was some kind of shameless cougar-wannabe.)

"Don't tell on me. *Please?*" I sounded like a kid who'd just broken her mom's favorite knickknack—except for where the knickknack might have been my skull.

He smiled, and it was all good.

We got through the nipple injection; I just stared into those baby blues and, under the theory of displacement of pain, focused on my aching head instead of the needle stabbing my boob. When we were done, he put his big, warm hand on my shoulder and told me I'd done a good job, a twinkle in his eye and a gentle look on his face.

Thank you, Dreamboat, for making a bad day better. And much, much funnier.

Another Side Story

This one is shorter and also funny. (And I was high when it happened, which at least gave me an excuse.)

I arrived the morning of my mastectomy prepared to say goodbye to my left breast forever. I was not prepared for delays that left me waiting no so patiently, nervous, and hangry and wondering when the hell we'd be getting the show on the road. Fortunately, my hubby (who, for the record, laughed harder at the bonking-my-head-in-front-of-Dreamboat story than anyone else) was there with me and, seeing my distress, he asked the nurses if there was anything they could do. There was.

I got some kind of relaxing medication in my IV that made me loopy, happy, and really friendly. I'm a happy drunk, hugging my friends and family while telling them and everyone else how much I love them, so it makes sense that I'm a happy high. The meds kicked in, and suddenly I was floating on a cloud, no longer hungry but very, very affectionate. According to hubby, I told him I loved him about twenty times, thanked everyone who came into the room for taking such great care of me, and asked about fifty times if I could call the kids.

He'd taken my phone away (!), saying he didn't want me "drunk texting" or "dropping the phone." Whatever. (I know it was just that he wanted my undivided attention so I could tell him, "I love you, man. Don't you know how much I *love* you?"[6])

By the time my surgeon—an insanely competent, no-nonsense, tough-yet-tender woman who normally wore cute dresses with kick-ass cowgirl boots (that I may or may not want to steal)—entered the room in scrubs, I was feeling no pain and a whole lot of euphoria. Maybe it was that I'd taken meds on an empty stomach, or maybe it was just me being me, but I looked at her with genuine awe and wonder as she talked us through the plan.

Just as she was exiting the room, I called out, "Dr. Meszoely?"

She turned and looked at me expectantly—probably thinking I was going to ask (another) off-the-wall question about tumor biology (*Here we go again*), if my colleague who'd asked for my tissue to make a new cell line could have it (*No, too late*), what they were going to do with my extra breast tissue and if I could have it for my lab work (*No*), or could I have her boots (*Definitely no*).

I took a deep breath, smiled, and said, "I love you."

She froze, looking confused and a little disturbed, while my husband sat in the corner, laughing his ass off. After a long, awkward pause, she said, "Um, I love you, too," and quickly exited the room.

I don't remember anything after that. I don't even remember waking up. I just remember asking for my phone (#Priorities) so I could call the kids and tell them I was okay. Apparently, I had already called the kids, and my daughter had been entertained by Drunk Mom. Hubby kissed my forehead, fed me dinner—bland steak and potatoes that were a far cry from the cheeseburger I'd asked him to smuggle into the hospital for when I woke up—and then left me to sleep it off.

I got my cheeseburger the next day, and when I followed up with Dr. Meszoely, I got a hug. (She loves me. She really, truly loves me!) Thanks, doc.

The Drag Queen and the Graduate Student: An Unlikely but Beautiful Love Story

This happened long before I was diagnosed with cancer, but it totally relates in my mind. I'll explain as we go. It'll all make sense by the end—I promise.

When I was in graduate school, in my mid-twenties, full of energy, anxiety, hopes, and dreams, and blessed with big, bouncy boobs that hadn't tried to kill me yet, getting out of the lab and blowing off steam by dancing at the Connection—the best (and only) gay bar I'd ever been to at this point in my young life—was my go-to.[7] (It was, IMHO, the best place to dance in Nashville in the 1990s.)

My impression of the Connection wasn't wrong. The forty-four thousand square feet of out-of-the-way, unused warehouse-style-space-turned-entertainment-venue-extravaganza boasted a patio and an enormous dance floor that allowed full-bodily expressions of joy and abandon fueled by fantastic music, strong cocktails, and the safety of knowing that no skeevy (straight) guys were likely to invade your space—and if they did, your friends and vigilant gay patrons would rescue you. I had grown up in the small and uber-conservative town of Maryville in East Tennessee, and my experience with the LGBT[8] community was limited to high school friends who were suspected but not out, ugly jokes told by the ignorant and bigoted, and whispered scandals about people suspected of being one of "those people" who would be doomed to the depths of Hell if they didn't get right with God.

Coming to Nashville was an awakening for me on many levels—not the least of which was learning to appreciate, love, and protect the beautiful rainbow people who brought magic to my life, my community, and the world. Four amazing gay fellow students were a large part of this awakening, friends who became like brothers, whom I still love and cherish to this day. They introduced me and other straight classmates to the wonders of the Connection. It was a place full of cowboys and angels, drag queens bedecked in glitter and glamor, and up to two thousand people dancing, reveling, and celebrating together in a sea of harmony, peace, and love.

And the music? It was a smorgasbord of '90s gay club anthems and diva house music—from CeCe Peniston and Crystal Waters to David Morales and Black Box—along with '80s ala Depeche Mode and Erasure. There was room to move and dance freely, thanks to the space, and you couldn't be self-conscious about your dance moves; someone was *always* doing something more outrageous or weirder than you were.

Yeah, there were drugs and casual hookups, and the hatred and intolerance of the outside world couldn't be kept completely at bay.[9] But that was a part of my awakening too. I learned that I am obliged, as a straight White woman of privilege, to be an active ally and work for justice and equality for my gay brothers and sisters in the alphabet mafia. We've come a long way since the '90s, but we still have a ways to go (more on this back in chapter 6).

One memorable night of clubbing, I volunteered to be designated driver for our Saturday night visit to the Connection. (Remember that. I was stone-cold sober for this encounter.)

I wasn't much for glamor, and my gays regularly coached me on how to be more fashionable and stylish—which was, sadly, an exercise in frustration. (For them. *I* was highly entertained.) Anyway, that night I wore a form-fitting pastel yellow short-sleeved mock-turtleneck sweater, jeans, and comfortable flats for dancing. My makeup was subtle. I could hardly hope to compete with the beauty and flawless flashiness of the drag queens we were going to see that night. We were going to what would be my first live drag show, and I was giddy as a schoolgirl.

I would learn that night what so many already knew: drag is an art form and drag queens are talented and dedicated performance artists who work hard to perfect their look, stage presence, and material.

What an extravaganza! So many sequined, rhinestoned, and be-dazzled outfits molding to the curves of glamorous queens sparkled from the stage as they danced, lip-synched, told jokes, and charmed the enthusiastic audience. Mere mortals like me basked in their glory and, on occasion, offered tips. As a reward, tippers received thank-yous, air kisses, winks, twirls, flirtations, and appreciation. That's what I ex-pected when I finally worked up the courage to approach the stage and tip one of the glorious creatures who had blown me away with her act and her dress—a much brighter shade of yellow that perfectly comple-mented her flawless black skin, including ample cleavage on display.

But that's not what I got.

My friends gay and straight cheered me on as I walked toward the stage, marveling at how much prettier the queen was as I got closer. Her contour game was perfect, giving her a round face with cheekbones that looked like they could cut glass. She looked at me, fluttering her long eyelashes to reveal sparkling eyeshadow and perfect liner, and pursed her red lips.

I'm guessing she recognized fresh meat when she saw me, blushing and giggling.

Meanwhile, I was wondering how she managed to balance in stilet-tos.

I held out my fiver and smiled. She bent slightly and accepted the bill, tucking it discreetly into her cleavage. Then, she looked at me—more specifically, my boobs—looked at her boobs, looked back at my boobs, looked at her boobs, cupped her boobs, and then reached down and cupped my boobs.

That's right. My friends, strangers, and half of gay Nashville watched me get felt up by a drag queen.

Okay, it *sounds* bad, but it didn't feel like a violation at the time or now. There was nothing sexual about it (she was, after all, looking for the same thing I was looking for—a man), and it wasn't an act of dominance or intimidation. She wasn't trying to humiliate me. She was just . . . comparing. And going for a laugh. Which she got. And though I was beet red and wondering how long it would take news of this little adventure to spread throughout my graduate school class, I laughed, too.

I laughed all the way back to my seat and enjoyed a chorus of applause. The funniest part? One of the faculty in my graduate program who was there that night snuck up behind my seat, tapped me on the shoulder, and, when I turned around, grinned wide and said, "I want to be on *your* thesis committee!"

I think about that night often and with fondness. To that beautiful drag queen, wherever you are, thank you for sharing your magic with me.

Little did that drag queen know, but a few decades later I would be getting an augmentation to my boobs' Spectacular Factor that would have left her and everyone at the Connection *speechless.*

Cancer: It'll Put Hair on Your Chest

It's interesting how autologous reconstruction after mastectomy (see chapter 4) rearranges your body in new and unexpected ways. My plastic surgeon took tissue from my right inner thigh and grafted it beneath the skin remaining from my mastectomy to build a new left breast. A small, triangular patch of skin from the donor-thigh tissue was attached to the native breast skin to finish up that part of the procedure.

When I woke up from surgery and had a look, I was impressed. Sure, the left breast was smaller than the right, but my surgeon assured me that with additional fat grafts during revision procedures he would be able to match the left breast to the right in terms of size and shape, and with massage we would be able to soften the tissue that had been damaged from radiation for a natural look and feel. I was (and am) on board, especially since I've seen significant improvement after the first revision/fat-grafting procedure (see chapter 16, figure 16.7).

I didn't pay too much attention to the undersides of my breasts after the initial graft in the first weeks after surgery. Other than changing gauze pads and other surgical dressings that covered the incisions, it was best to leave well enough alone until the site had a chance to heal. And they healed beautifully! Once I had the green light from my surgeon, I started massaging my left breast to soften the tissue in preparation for the first revision.

That's when I felt it: Hair. *Lots* of hair.

The patch of skin from my donor thigh was covered with soft, dark hair that had reached an impressive length six weeks after surgery. We're talking at least an inch, if not more. It was *freaky*. I could tug it, twist it, and, with the aid of a mirror, probably could have braided it. I considered dying it neon blue or some other cool color, figuring I could hop on the trend train with all of those ladies growing out, coloring, and bedazzling their armpit hair. (Hubby vetoed that idea.[10])

What's a hairy-boobed lady to do?

Laugh, of course. I almost fell off the bed laughing when I discovered my new pelt. And why not? Celebrating life and new boobs-in-progress, with all of their weirdness, sparked an odd kind of joy and a new appreciation for the wonders of the human body—my human body—on its journey to wholeness.

I laugh in the face of cancer.

And Speaking of Medicine . . .

So, I'll bet you've run across advertisements for supplements, essential oils, fad diets, and other products that make out-of-this-world claims about the health benefits of whatever they're peddling. Ever hear a chiropractor claim they've cured diseases? I have. What about the effects of essential oils on general wellness? Sure. How about *Cannabis is the cure for cancer, but the government/big pharma doesn't want you to know?* Oh, that's a big one on Facebook.

These claims are false, but peddlers are getting more devious and clever with their advertising—like sneaking in links to genuine, peer-reviewed studies to make it seem like legitimate scientific data supports the spurious product claims, but on closer inspection it totally doesn't.

How can you tell what's real and what's a big, steaming pile of *bullshit*?

I'll give you some tips in the next chapter.

~

PART III

SCIENCE SAVVY

Why You Should Listen to Your Doctor
and Not Dave "Avocado" Wolfe,
Gwyneth Paltrow, or Darla Shine

CHAPTER TEN

~

Avoid the Woo! How to Spot Scams and Distinguish Pseudoscience from What's Legit When It Comes to Breast Cancer

What do David "Avocado" Wolfe, Gwyneth Paltrow, and Darla Shine have in common? They all have exploited the popularity of the "alternative medicine" and "wellness" movements in our culture to peddle woo. What is *woo*? It's another name for bullshit scams for health and wellness that have no scientific or medical basis but are marketed as an alternative to conventional medicine, while medicine is often described as "unnatural" or part of a conspiracy to keep people in the dark about "real" and "natural" cures for what ail them.

At best, woo is a scam that robs people of their hard-earned cash. At worst, it can be deadly.

Note: I'm not lumping complementary alternative medicine into the woo category. *Complementary alternative medicine* is just what it sounds like: It is the combination of conventional, standard-of-care, effective therapies with alternative therapies that haven't been tested or scientifically vetted or that *have* been tested but have not been shown to be effective. So long as the alternative medicine doesn't interfere with proven therapies, I say go for it. Like essential oils? Use them! Aromatherapy won't hurt you (unless you're allergic to florals or other ingredients). Just don't skip your chemotherapy or other treatments because you think essential oils will cure your cancer. They won't. Does acupuncture help you with pain management? Do it! But don't skip out on physical therapy or other measures your health-care team prescribes. These types of alternative therapies can provide comfort. Massage and reflexology, meditation and mindfulness (those two have some solid research behind them[1]), Reiki and homeopathy (homeopathy has been disproven,[2] and Reiki is arguably a spiritual practice, which, like other spiritual and religious practices, relies on faith rather than rigorous testing)—these all can help ease stress and give patients a sense of well-being. They may even elicit a *placebo effect*—a phenomenon in which some patients experience a benefit from the control substance (like a sugar pill or dummy pill) that has no known medical effect. The power of belief may be behind this effect as applied to complementary alternative therapies.[3]

But complementary alternative therapies are no replacement for clinically proven cancer treatments. Some forms of complementary medicine won't hurt you, but they reportedly produce *no benefit in terms of survival.*[4] A study specific to breast cancer also reports no survival benefit for complementary alternative medicine.[5]

Do inform your health-care team about any complementary alternative therapies you're trying so they can make certain that these alternatives don't interfere with your prescribed medications or therapies.

Now, on to "alternative medicine" of the noncomplementary variety. These are the woo scams that make false claims of efficacy, attack standard-of-care proven medical practices with wild conspiracy theories to bolster their claims, and often play upon the fears and desperation of cancer patients for money. The Internet and social media have made it ridiculously easy for people with no medical or scientific training or without any relevant expertise to spread false claims and sell dubious and often dangerous products and practices. We live in an age of fake news and pseudoscience, made worse by the pervasive anti-intellectual and anti-science political culture gripping the United States and much of the world. From the anti-vax movement to conspiracy theories surrounding COVID-19, mistrust of science and medicine has gripped broad swaths of the US population, and unfortunately this mistrust extends to standard-of-care cancer treatments and cancer biology.

I have very strong feelings about these scams and the people and corporations that pedal them, and I have covered a few of these on my blog,[6] separating fact from fiction when it comes to turmeric, apple cider vinegar, essential oils, and antioxidants. In this chapter, I'll cover cannabis, products and practices peddled by Gwyneth Paltrow's company Goop, self-proclaimed wellness guru David "Avocado" Wolfe, and Darla Shine, wife of former White House communications director Bill Shine, who likes to use Twitter to spread anti-science nonsense. By debunking their bogus claims with actual peer-reviewed science, my hope is to show you how to put on your skeptic hat and look for red flags so you too can learn to identify the too-good-to-be-true modern-day snake-oil "cures" and can protect your health *and* your wallet.

Why do I have a bug up my butt about this issue? A recent study from *Journal of the National Cancer Institute* tracked patients with curable cancer who opted out of conventional therapies and relied on "alternative medicine." Sadly, compared to patients with similar cancers of comparable stage and grade who *did* complete conventional therapies, patients who relied on alternative medicine had worse outcomes—meaning many of them died. The study controlled for other independent clinical and demographic factors.[7] Even I—who work in the field—was shocked and appalled to read that most of the alternative-medicine crowd in this study were more likely to be comprised of young women with higher education and income and who had received a diagnosis of a higher cancer stage. Women—my sisters—presumably with access to scientifically accurate information, with greater financial means, and at higher risk for death from their cancers opted to put their faith in unproven treatments, and many of them died unnecessarily because of it. Moreover, many of these alternatives cause harm in and of themselves.

We have *got* to do better than this, be better, and fight the woo.

Let's start with cannabis. *Cannabis sativa*, *Cannabis indica*, and *Cannabis ruderalis* are some of the many varieties of this plant that has such a sordid history in the United States. Marijuana, weed, ganja, pot, grass, reefer, dope, Mary Jane, and hash—it's most associated with recreational illegal drug use. Legalization in several states and the commercialization of cannabis production are giving cannabis a PR makeover, as is increasing interest in its medicinal uses. Beyond the psychoactive ingredient delta-9-tetrahydrocannabinol (THC), which produces the high, cannabidiol (CBD) has become a popular "natural" treatment for pain, anxiety and depression, acne, neurological disorders like epilepsy and multiple sclerosis, high blood pressure, and chemotherapy-induced nausea and vomiting in cancer patients.[8] Though more research is necessary—and will hopefully become easier with legalization—evidence for these benefits is promising. In fact, commercially available synthetic THC (dronabinol and nabilone) has been approved for treatment of cancer-*related* side effects,[9] not to be confused with cancer treatment.

Currently, in order to conduct a clinical trial with botanical cannabis in the United States, investigators need to get a Schedule I license from the US Drug Enforcement Administration and approval from the National Institute on Drug Abuse, a process that is difficult, time-consuming, and largely cost prohibitive. That's a shame, because the medicinal value of this plant has been recognized for millennia, and removing legal barriers and the social stigma surrounding it could uncover benefits not only from THC and CBD but from other cannabinoids that have been underinvestigated as well.

But the waters get murky when it comes to cannabis and its die-hard fans and proponents who make wild and unsubstantiated claims about the drug's medicinal uses.

What's disturbing? The rise in false claims, largely shared on social media platforms, that cannabis is a cure for cancer. According to Shi et al., cannabis as a cancer cure represented 23.5 percent of social media content from 2017 to 2018, with reader engagement that dwarfed engagement with accurate news stories debunking false claims. Also, they report that cancer organizations rarely address the actual limits of cannabis's efficacy, failing to provide information to refute false claims.[10] False claims are often bolstered by conspiracy theories, such as the popular but inaccurate claim that big pharma is suppressing evidence of cannabis cures because it threatens their profits from expensive cancer treatments. The government is probably "in" on it too, according to conspiracy theorists.[11] I spend way too much time on Facebook arguing with strangers, and I've been accused of being a pharma shill when I've dared to challenge conspiracy-theory posts. *Note:* I've tested experimental drugs in collaboration with pharmaceutical companies, but I've never received those fabled big payouts for my work. Hell, one fool even claimed that I used conventional therapy for my own cancer treatments in order to keep the "big secret" about the cannabis cure.

Talk about taking one for the team!! If there was a cure and I knew about it, not only would I *take* it, but I would also be shouting about it from the rooftops and into all corners of the Internet.

But, as we discussed in chapter 2, cancer is a complex collection of adaptable diseases and is quite difficult to cure, and one cure won't likely fit all cancers because of their diversity at the molecular and genetic levels.

So, has cannabis been tested as a potential treatment for cancer— and by that I mean in a clinical trial and not the kind of testing my cousin used to do with the plants he grew himself?

One ongoing trial is testing the effect of different types of cannabis and cannabinoids on quality of life for stage II to IV non-small-cell lung cancer patients.[12] This study is designed to test medical benefits including anti-nausea and -vomiting effects, appetite stimulation, pain relief, and improved sleep. Notice that the trial *doesn't* include antitumor effects as an end point. Why? Most likely because preclinical studies conducted in laboratory models have been contradictory or inconclusive. I'll summarize.[13]

Several studies of cannabis in laboratory mouse and rat cancer models suggest antitumor effects in liver cancer, breast cancer, brain cancer, and lung cancer and suggest protection from chemically induced malignancies in colon cancer, as well as showing antimetastasis effects in some of these laboratory rodent models. CBD might enhance cancer-cell uptake of chemotherapeutic agents in mouse models, importantly *without* affecting normal cells. However, bear in mind that these animal models are immunocompromised, meaning they lack a lot of the natural disease-fighting machinery a normal animal would have. This allows scientists to graft human tumor cells into the animals to study the effects of drugs, but it leaves out a part of normal physiology that plays a huge role in tumor biology (see more in chapter 16). That's an important consideration, especially since two studies using immunocompetent mouse models with intact, fully functional immune systems reported immunosuppressive effects and enhanced tumor growth.

What does it all mean? *Bottom line:* cannabis and two of its active components, THC and CBD, can benefit cancer patients by helping fight the nasty side effects of chemotherapy and other treatments. Preclinical studies on the antitumor effects need a *lot* of work, better

144 ~ Chapter Ten

models, and reproducibility studies (this is true for much of cancer research) before clinical testing can begin, which won't likely happen until legal barriers are removed. Will cannabis alone cure your cancer? *No, it won't.*

Please don't rely on cannabis alone. I am begging you.

Next up, let's talk about Goop, actress Gwyneth Paltrow's "wellness and lifestyle brand and company." Lots of people shit on Gwyneth Paltrow. Personally, I adore her as an actress. I'm a Marvel Cinematic Universe gal and enjoyed her as Pepper Potts. I also enjoyed *Shakespeare in Love,* and both my husband and I laughed out loud when we watched *View from the Top.* It has been reported that Paltrow supports the American Cancer Society, the Breast Cancer Research Foundation, the Dana-Farber Cancer Institute, the Melanoma Research Alliance, Stand Up to Cancer, and the Women's Cancer Research Fund.[14] When it comes to health and wellness advice doled out by an entertainer, however, I'll listen to Dr. Ken Jeong, who actually has a medical degree (and is freaking hilarious in film and stand-up) rather than Ms. Paltrow. What's wrong with Gwyneth Paltrow using her celebrity status to make a buck? Nothing—*if* it were restricted to supporting products that did not make false claims about the health benefits of overpriced weird shit, like vagina eggs and vaginal steaming. (And the whole "this candle smells like my vagina" thing is super weird.)[15]

At least Goop got called out and penalized for false claims about the jade vagina eggs—specifically bogus claims that they "increase vaginal muscle tone, hormonal balance, and feminine energy in general." Goop settled a consumer-protection lawsuit out of court for $145,000 for the company's false claims related to jade eggs, rose quartz eggs, and an essential-oil blend.[16] Dr. Jen Gunter, OB/GYN and author of *The Vagina Bible* (which I highly recommend reading), thoroughly debunks vagina eggs with peer-reviewed science and medicine in a thoroughly entertaining way and also reminds women *not* to steam their vaginas— another practice endorsed by Paltrow and Goop.[17] (Seriously, don't steam your vajazzle. Yeast infections are terribly uncomfortable, as are vulval burns.)

What does Goop have to do with cancer? Turns out, "experts" featured on her Netflix show, *The Goop Lab,* have made false claims about the effects of their practices on cancer. John Amaral, "somatic energy practitioner" (a bullshit term for something that doesn't actually exist), not only claims that he healed a woman of her knee pain just before her scheduled surgery, but also implied that he could make breast cancer disappear. The transcript from a 2018 interview with Stephan Spencer published by *Vice* quotes Amaral:

> Many things are possible. Cancers can be gone in an instant. I've had patients that I've worked with where they had been diagnosed with breast cancer. They were on my table, and there was a shift. They felt themselves shifting to a different reality where that nodule was gone. They looked for it, and it's gone. They would go in, get tested, and it's not there. They're like, "What happened?" Spontaneous remission. They literally flipped, in my experience, into a different version of themselves. In that reality, they did not have cancer. I've experienced things like this many times working with people. It's been validated by testing and science.[18]

As you might expect, this has most certainly *not* been validated by testing and science. It actually reminds me of faith healing—the laying on of hands that charlatans pretending to be preachers use to heal true believers . . . for a fee. Don't fall for it. Mr. Amaral is no different than other snake-oil salesmen out to make a buck off desperate people. Before his appearance on *The Goop Lab*, he added one-on-one sessions for the bargain price of $2,500 to his website and is seeking to trademark his Energy Flow Formula for the treatment of various illnesses.[19] Sure, he includes legal disclaimers on his website, but if he didn't make spurious claims, he wouldn't have to.

Goop also published a piece by a so-called "expert" who claims underwire bras might cause breast cancer (they don't[20]). The blog post was written by a PhD in classical studies (not cancer biology or another relevant field) about what to do following a cancer diagnosis and supports "Gerson Therapy," which involves a specific organic vegetarian diet, supplements, and enemas to treat cancer (there's no scientific evidence to support this "treatment" for cancer[21]).

What does it all mean? *Bottom line:* Goop and Gwyneth Paltrow are definitely not the sources you should go to for advice on cancer treatments. The approaches they endorse range from bizarre to dangerous and will cost you a pretty penny. I agree with Dr. Victoria Forster, cancer researcher and cancer survivor: Gwyneth Paltrow's Goop should stay in its lane, far away from people with cancer.[22]

Quick note: If you're a cancer survivor looking for a good source a good source of information on healthy eating, my medical oncologist, Dr. Brent Rexer, offers a lot of good suggestions on his blog, Feasting on Veggies.[23] Part of his ongoing research involves looking at how diet could alter tumor metabolism, including the activity of proteins that drive cancer and are drug targets. Again, trust your health-care providers, and tap them for information instead of relying on information peddled by a celebrity with no medical training.

Next up is one of my least favorite people in the whole wide world, David "Avocado" Wolfe. As Yvette d'Entremont—aka SciBabe, aka one of my heroes, who's taken on the mantle of protecting the world from pseudoscience—puts it, "David Avocado Wolfe is the biggest asshole in the multiverse."[24] She's not wrong. Why? He is a notorious anti-vaxxer, believes in chemtrails,[25] and peddles all kinds of crazy woo crap on a variety of dubious websites and Facebook. You've probably come across some of his memes and bullshit claims on social media. Since SciBabe covers a multitude of his false claims and debunks them, as does Dan Broadbent (aka A Science Enthusiast),[26] I'm going to focus specifically on his spurious cancer claims and debunk them.

Looking for an alternative medicine to treat your cancer? Avocado Boy claims that you need look no further than vitamin B-17 (the synthetic version is called laetrile), even going so far as to cite a so-called cancer researcher-expert from a prestigious cancer-research institution.[27] Oddly enough, Wolfe doesn't provide links to scientific research published by this expert or any others to back up his claim. Hmm . . . As if that weren't enough of a red flag, a quick Google search led me to Cancer Research UK's website and an article stating not only that there is no scientific research backing claims that laetrile can treat cancer but also that laetrile contains cyanide![28] Please, please, please do not ingest a deadly poison that can kill you—which defeats the whole purpose of cancer treatment.

But what else would you expect from a charlatan? I'll tell you: claims that mushrooms can fight cancer. According to another blog post I'm loath to link, chaga mushroom supplements can reduce cancer growth.[29] What's the evidence? Apparently, some active ingredient in

Vaccines are safe. They do not cause autism. They. Do. Not. Cause. Autism. We've spent billions of dollars proving the safety of vaccines, largely because one greedy douchecanoe named Andrew Wakefield—who was stripped of his medical license for fraud—falsified data linking the MMR vaccine to autism in a really shitty study sponsored by lawyers for parents involved in lawsuits with vaccine manufacturers.[a] The study originally published in *The Lancet* was retracted. Wakefield never replicated his alleged findings, and neither has he ever admitted he was wrong, unlike ten of his coauthors who publicly denounced the validity of the "data." In fact, this guy still has followers. He's still out there fueling the anti-vax movement and profiting from it, now using his dubious clout to spread lies about the SARS-CoV-2/ COVID-19 vaccines.[b] He should be put in a stockade and left to be jeered at while facing the families of every single person who has died because of the anti-vax movement he spawned, as well as by every person with autism and their family, on whom the money wasted debunking his false claims could have been used for legitimate autism research and interventions.

Sources:

a. Fiona Godlee, Jane Smith, and Harvey Marcovitch, "Wakefield's Article Linking MMR Vaccine and Autism Was Fraudulent," *BMJ* 342 (January 5, 2011): c7452, https://doi.org/10.1136/bmj.c7452, https:// www.ncbi.nlm.nih.gov/pubmed/21209060.

b. Peter Jamison, "Anti-vaccination Leaders Sieze on Coronavirus to Push Resistance to Inoculation," Social Issues, *Washington Post*, May 5, 2020, https://www.washingtonpost.com/dc-md-va/2020/05/05/anti- vaxxers-wakefield-coronavirus-vaccine/.

the mushroom kills cancer cell lines in a petri dish (we've been killing cancer cells in culture for decades with agents that unfortunately didn't work in humans) and in inbred mice with transplanted tumors treated with the mushroom supplement in drinking water. These studies show up in databases curating peer-reviewed research. But dig a little deeper, and you'll see why this is problematic. First of all, the mouse study[30] doesn't look for or measure any active ingredient from the mushroom in the bloodstream or tumor tissue of treated mice, which is pharmacokinetics 101. If you think something has an effect on disease, you study how it is metabolized and whether or not it even makes it to the diseased tissue. Probably not a bad idea to know what protein or proteins it binds to and what molecular pathways it affects (that's sarcasm). You should *totally* investigate the molecular mechanism and make it a part of your study. Plus, if you know what pathways your mushroom goo affects, you can see if those pathways are altered in human cancer samples to lend what we call *clinical relevance* to your study.

What does it all mean? *Bottom line:* don't take advice from self-proclaimed wellness gurus. Granted, his blog post on mushrooms does cite scientific literature[31] (though with an impact factor of 0.432, *Helioyn* isn't publishing the best studies; for comparison, *Cancer Research*, one of the most respected cancer journals, has an impact factor of 9.130; that's not to say it's a "bad" study, just not particularly rigorous or impactful) and even clarifies that the studies cited are from cell culture and animal models. But he still implies that mushrooms have health benefits for humans and will gladly sell you his products: "To harness these and other mushroom benefits, check out our mushroom powders and mushroom tinctures."[32] We'll discuss this a bit more in the next chapter on how to get the real scoop behind headlines, but cell culture and animal studies *do not* prove that a supplement or alternative therapy will work in humans. You need clinical trials performed in humans for that, and the evidence linked in the mushroom study in mouse cancer models is not nearly enough to support a trial in humans.

And I say that as a basic science researcher who uses mouse models and cell-culture studies all the time. They're essential for working out the cell biology and molecular and genetic mechanisms that drive cancer, and when studied in detail and linked to human cancers using clinical data, basic research in laboratory models can provide a strong rationale for testing new therapies in clinical trials. But you have to be thorough and comprehensive, and you have to test new therapies rigorously in these models first.

The last example I'll cover is Darla Shine. Hers is an . . . interesting case of combining anti-vax crap with the false claim that having measles as a child protects against cancer later in life. This is a really terrible twofer, since her nonsense coincides with measles outbreaks in the United States and Europe (thanks, anti-vaxxers) and spreads preposterous bullshit about an alleged protective effect that a nearly eradicated disease (prior to the anti-vax movement) has on cancer. Like all of the cool kids, rather than sharing her discoveries in peer-reviewed scientific or medical journals, Darla chooses to spread the word on Twitter. In response to a CNN report linking the anti-vax movement to recent measles outbreaks, she tweeted, "Here we go LOL #measlesoutbreak on CNN #fake #hysteria. The entire Baby Boom population alive today had the #Measles as kids. Bring back our #ChildhoodDiseases they keep you healthy & fighting cancer."[33]

Maybe she should ask the baby boom generation if they remember friends crippled by polio and how their parents lined up to make sure they got their polio vaccines. Remember iron lungs?[34] No, you probably don't, *because the polio vaccine wiped out this horrible virus in the United States by 1979.*[35]

Is there evidence for an anticancer effect produced by a measles infection? Nope. But Darla maintains via Twitter that "I had the measles, that was the whole point of my tweet. I have life time [sic] natural immunity."[36] This little anecdote brings up the important distinction between *correlation* and *causality*. I love Khan Academy, so let's visit it for an explanation of each of these terms and the distinction between the two.

According to Khan Academy, "*correlation* means there is a relationship or pattern between the values of two variables."[37] For example, smoking correlates with the incidence of lung cancer. Does that prove that smoking causes lung cancer? No. In order to prove causality—which means that one event causes another to happen—you need to perform appropriately designed experiments. It took decades of research, not to mention fighting the tobacco industry, to prove the causal link between carcinogens in cigarette smoke and DNA damage that leads to malignant transformation of lung cells.[38] In order for Darla to test her "hypothesis" that measles protects against cancer later in life—based on her "observational study" of herself, apparently—she would need to conduct epidemiological studies to track cancer cases in people who have had measles during childhood and those who have not. Assuming she found some kind of correlation, she would need to perform studies in laboratory models and work out the molecular mechanism(s) through which the measles virus stops cancer a long time after infection.

Of course, in order to do any of that Darla would need to earn a degree in biological sciences or medicine, complete clinical-research training, and convince an institution to sponsor her study as well as get research funding.

Darla has yet to do this.

Suffice to say, *there is no evidence that measles has an anticancer effect,* but interestingly enough Darla may have gotten the idea from legitimate studies conducted by actual scientists using *engineered* versions of the measle virus to infect and kill cancer cells and to induce antitumor immunity. The team of investigators behind this legitimate research wrote a whole article about what their research does and does not show in order to address anti-vaxxers and people like our friend Darla. I'll let them speak for themselves:

> Vaccination protects against measles and has been administered to over a billion people with an exceptional safety record. There is no evidence that measles infection can protect against cancer. Our studies using engineered measles viruses to treat cancer have found the best outcomes in people who have been vaccinated, and our current approaches are fully geared to this group of patients with cancer.
>
> We are dismayed to learn that our work is being cited in opposition to MMR (measles, mumps, and rubella) vaccination and are therefore taking this opportunity to review the key pertinent facts about measles, measles vaccination, and measles as an experimental cancer therapy that support this position.[39]

They go on to note that there is *no evidence* that natural measles infection can protect against cancer later in life. The research they are conducting involves an attenuated (meaning weakened by laboratory methods and unable to cause disease) measles strain to kill cancer cells, including viruses engineered to deliver anticancer genes to enhance tumor-cell killing and other modifications that direct the engineered virus to selectively attack cancer cells.[40] It's a clever, elegant strategy that is currently being tested in humans, but, as noted, the virus the investigators are using as a delivery tool is *far* removed from the natural measles virus.

What does it all mean? *Bottom line:* don't skip your kiddos' measles vaccine in hopes of saving them from cancer. Don't be like Darla. Dig deep into the science, and ask your health-care providers to guide you so you can get the full scoop, accurate information, and avoid being duped.

How do you protect yourself from scams like these? The American Cancer Society provides a great list of red flags that will help you discern scientifically sound advice from pseudoscience woo:

1. Beware claims that an alternative treatment can cure cancer.
2. Beware claims that a treatment can offer benefits without side effects. If the treatment is reported to have no side effects, it has likely not been tested in clinical trials where side effects would be seen and documented.
3. Beware alternative medicine peddlers who attack scientists and medical providers or who tell you that you should avoid standard-of-care treatments. Conspiracy-theory central. Don't fall for it.
4. Beware "exclusive" therapies that you can get in only one clinic, especially if that clinic is in a country with less-strict patient-protection laws than those in the United States, Canada, the United Kingdom, or the European Union.
5. Look out for red-flag terms such as "scientific breakthrough," "miracle cure," "secret ingredient," or "ancient remedy." Don't trust personal stories or anecdotes that claim amazing results but fail to provide scientific evidence to back them up.
6. Check the credentials of anyone advising you about an alternative treatment. Find out if they're actually medical doctors and/ or experts in cancer care or complementary medicines. Don't trust chiropractors.
7. Do your research to see if peer-reviewed scientific studies or clinical trials have been conducted for the treatment in people (not just animal models) and to learn which side effects have been reported. Check with your health-care team to see if the alterna-

tive treatment could hurt you or interact with other medicines or supplements you are taking.

8. Check peer-reviewed, scientific literature (published in trustworthy journals, like those curated in PubMed database[41]) for information on the safety and effectiveness of treatments. Beware treatments only promoted in the mass media—like books, magazines, the Internet, TV, infomercials, and radio talk shows. Don't waste your money on crap sold by Alex Jones, Goop, or David Avocado Wolfe.[42]

As we'll see in the next chapter, this list of red flags will also help you evaluate the trustworthiness of news reports related to science. I'll show you how to look past sensational headlines that are great for selling ads but not so good for disseminating accurate information and aren't much more than clickbait.

There are lots of really amazing, newsworthy discoveries being made every day in the field of cancer research. Together we'll go through some examples to help you learn how to get to the heart of the story in its proper context and uncover what the discovery really means.

~

CHAPTER ELEVEN

How to Look Past the Sensational Headlines and Get the Real Scoop from Science Reporting

When I was in graduate school, I got a lot of questions: *What exactly do you do? When are you going to graduate? Why didn't you just get a real job and start making money?*

Answers included, *I'm doing very important work as a scientist, following the noble calling of disease research, looking for cures* (read: I'm desperately trying to remind myself why the hell I'm in lab at midnight repeating an experiment I already fucked up twice this week instead of chucking it all and playing the lottery to underwrite my lavish lifestyle). *I'm going to graduate soon. Like, I just have a couple more experiments and a paper to publish, and I'm totally there. Really. This time I mean it* (read: I'm never getting out of here. I'm going to be a lacky, barely paid intern/indentured servant in the academic machine forever). As for why I didn't just get a real job and start making money, see answer number one.

One of the other questions that came from family, (nonscience) friends, and sometimes people at bars started out with, "Hey, I read a newspaper article/Facebook post that said someone's cured cancer. Did you hear about that?"

This is the particular question that inspired this chapter and one that never fails to make my ass twitch with irritation. Look—there's nothing I'd love more than to be out of a job because someone out there finds cures for all cancers, but as I have already said in earlier chapters, that ain't likely to happen anytime soon. I'm not blaming nonscientists for not knowing everything going on in Science at large, and I think science journalists are doing the best they can within a media system that values sensation and buzz (which leads to more advertising dollars) over balanced headlines. My goal with this chapter is to share some tips on how you can discern the truth behind the headlines and interpret what the scientific study reported on actually shows.

Why? Because I *do* blame scientists (myself included) for failing to inform the public about what they do. By and large, we're introverts. We're nerds. We love to talk nerdy shit with each other. But ask us to talk to someone who has never held a test tube?

Most of us are stumped or terrified.

We need to get over it. Given the increasingly science- and technology-driven society in which we live, where direct-to-consumer advertising tells us (sort of) about some drug that "might be right for you" but doesn't tell us what the hell the drug is for or how it works, where we're all getting a crash course in virology thanks to SARS-CoV-2, the nasty little virus responsible for the global COVID pandemic, and where terms like "gene editing" and "mRNA vaccines" and "immune-checkpoint inhibitors" are bandied about without much explanation, scientists really need to work on outreach and spreading scientific literacy to the public. I mean, it's always great to get press coverage for scientific advances. It keeps the public informed and engaged, which leads to more interest and (hopefully) increased funding for laboratory and clinical investigation. But the news media gets stuff wrong, and that's *terrible* PR for science. Inaccurate reportage does little to keep the public informed and even less for public perception and expectations, especially when it comes to complex diseases like cancer. So scientists need to step up their communication game.

After all, most of us receive some form of federal funding for our research, which comes from tax dollars. I personally feel obligated to be able to explain what I do and why it is important in terms that can be understood by my mom, my kid, my nonscience friends, and anyone who asks. Knowledge is power, and taxpayers are funding the pursuit of knowledge. The public has the right to know what we're up to.

So, let's get to it.

I covered how to analyze and interpret science news related to cancer research on my blog,[1] and we'll dig deeper into this subject in a second. But since I don't want to get sued by an angry media conglomerate, I'm instead going to write up a few of mock articles based on my own work as examples. These will incorporate the common problems I've seen in actual science reporting and will hopefully help you hone your savvy interpretation skills.

I'll use a real paper I coauthored as the subject of these mock news articles: "Targeting EphA2 Impairs Cell Cycle Progression and Growth of Basal-like/Triple-Negative Breast Cancers." It was published in *Oncogene* in 2017,[2] and I'm pretty proud of it. Here's a quick summary: We mined mRNA-expression data from public databases and found out that levels of mRNA-encoding EphA2—a cell-surface receptor we study that tells cancer cells to grow and move—are really high in the basal-like, triple-negative breast cancer subtype (TNBC), as well as in the HER2+ subtype of human breast cancers. Using mouse models and cell-culture models, we found that blocking EphA2 expression reduced cell division and tumor growth in mice and in cells grown in culture dishes. We worked out a molecular pathway that linked EphA2 to cell-cycle driver pathways and showed that a pharmacologic inhibitor also blocked tumor growth in mice, which included specialized models called patient-derived xenografts (PDX). These models use patient tumor tissue transplanted directly into mice, and the tumor tissue behaves like it did in the original patient in terms of growth, metastasis, and drug responses.[3]

So, let's pretend that a science reporter got really excited about this paper we published and decided to write an article about it. The headline might read, "STUDY IDENTIFIES NEW TARGET FOR TREATING TRIPLE-NEGATIVE BREAST CANCER." Below the headline, the reporter might note, "New research finds that blocking a cell-surface receptor stops tumor growth in mice with triple-negative breast cancer by stopping cell-cycle progression." That's pretty accurate reporting. It tells us that the study was conducted in animal models and gives us a quick summary of the major findings—that blocking a cell-surface receptor in triple-negative breast tumors stops tumors from growing in laboratory mice by affecting the cell cycle.

The article might go on to report that

EphA2, a cell-surface receptor that is overexpressed in breast cancers across subtypes, may be a new drug target for triple-negative breast cancer (TNBC), an aggressive form of breast cancer that can currently only be treated with chemotherapy.[a] Breast cancer cells make more EphA2, and the investigators found that TNBC and HER2+ breast cancer, another aggressive subtype, have the highest levels of EphA2. When they blocked EphA2 gene expression in mice with TNBC, tumors stopped growing. Blocking EphA2 reduced levels of cell-cycle driver oncogene c-Myc[b] and elevated cell-cycle inhibitor p27/KIP1[c] in TNBC cells.[d] This stops tumor cells from dividing by blocking the transition from the growth phase of the cell to the DNA-synthesis phase of the cell cycle during which tumor cells replicate their DNA, known as the G_1 to S transition. A chemical inhibitor of EphA2 produced similar results.

To determine if their findings were relevant to human TNBC, the investigators found that high levels of EphA2 gene expression in TNBC patients were associated with reduced recurrence-free survival. High protein levels of EphA2 also positively correlated with high protein levels of c-Myc and low levels of p27/KIP1. These data match data produced in laboratory models.

TNBC represents approximately 10 to 15 percent of all breast cancers diagnosed. TNBCs lacks hormone receptors and the HER2 protein, which are targets for anticancer drugs. These breast cancers grow and metastasize faster, spreading to other parts of the patient's body, and have a worse prognosis than other types of breast cancer. Further research on EphA2 in TNBC is needed before drugs can be developed and tested in human clinical trials, including laboratory trials combining EphA2 blockers with chemotherapy or other drugs that might maximize tumor cell killing.

a. "Triple-Negative Breast Cancer," American Cancer Society medical and editorial content team, American Cancer Society, Cancer.org, last revised January 27, 2021, https://www.cancer.org/cancer/breast-cancer/understanding-a-breast-cancer-diagnosis/types-of-breast-cancer/triple-negative.html.

b. For more on the myc gene, see Faith Parsons, "Myc Gene Faith Parsons," video, YouTube, uploaded January 22, 2019, https://www.youtube.com/watch?v=e3tN-WVUSa8.

c. Neural Academy, "Cyclins and CDKs Cell Cycle Regulation," video, YouTube, uploaded May 1, 2018, https://www.youtube.comwatch?v=nEMMKzYQf9A.

d. For more on cell cycle and cancer, see AMBOSS, "Cell Cycle and Cancer: Phases, Hallmarks, and Development," video, YouTube, uploaded April 27, 2018, https://www.youtube.com/watch?v=e0lNk-2Il_M.

This (fictional) news report has all of the elements that I as a scientist would look for in a great news article about a scientific study: a citation for the study and a link to the publicly available article; background information plus links to literature or media with information about EphA2, c-Myc, p27/KIP1, and cell cycle; and background information plus links with information about TNBC.

It's helpful if reporters provide a link to the original study via an open-access version of the paper so they don't get stuck behind a paywall. Subscriptions to academic journals are crazy expensive, and even purchasing a single article can be pricey. But since most biomedical research is federally funded—at least in part—the National Institutes of Health mandate that a version of any manuscript funded by the NIH must be made publicly available after publication. You can find these versions at PubMed Central.[4]

Let's look at another example of how the same study might be covered by the news. The headline might read, "STUDY LINKS CELL-SURFACE RECEPTOR TO CANCER." It's somewhat vague. What kind of cancer? What kind of study? It's not bad per se, but compared to the headline in the first example, this one just isn't as specific. Things may become a bit more clear by the first sentence in the story: "A new study identifies a potential new target for treating triple-negative breast cancer." This tells us the study is related to triple-negative breast cancer, but it doesn't tell us that it's a laboratory study using mouse models. Again, this isn't bad reportage per se, but if you're skimming the news and only looking at headlines and a bit of the article, you might think the study was from human trials.

The article might go on to report,

A new study links EphA2 to growth of triple-negative breast cancer (TNBC), an aggressive form of breast cancer that can currently only be treated with chemotherapy. These breast cancer cells make more EphA2, and the investigators found that TNBC and HER2+ breast cancer, another aggressive subtype, have the highest levels of EphA2. When they blocked EphA2 function in laboratory mouse models of

TNBC, it stopped tumor growth in its tracks by blocking cell division. The researchers discovered that high levels of EphA2 gene expression in TNBC patients were associated with reduced recurrence-free survival, which may make EphA2 a good target for new cancer-fighting drugs. This is important, since TNBC, while occurring less frequently than other types of breast cancer, grows and spreads faster. Patients diagnosed with TNBC have a worse prognosis.

This reporting has fewer elements that I as a scientist would look for in a great news article about a scientific study: no citation for the study, and no link to the publicly available article; some background information, but no links to literature or media with information about EphA2; and background information on TNBC, but no links.

Also, in this version of news reportage on my paper, the fact that the study was conducted in animal models is mentioned late in the article. It isn't necessarily *inaccurate* that "the researchers discovered that high levels of EphA2 gene expression in TNBC patients were associated with reduced recurrence-free survival, which may make EphA2 a good target for new cancer fighting drugs," but the wording implies that we're close to testing EphA2-targeting drugs in human trials, which wasn't the case at the time of the article's publication.

Side note: Bicycle Therapeutics has an EphA2-targeting drug[5] in early clinical trials now, which is awesome, and I'm working with them to see if patients with residual or recurrent disease after HER2-targeted therapy may be good candidates to test the effectiveness of this drug. Recruitment for that clinical trial started in November of 2019,[6] two years after publication of our study.

This isn't a bad news article per se, but it would be so much better with links, more details about the findings in the context of laboratory models, and more clarity about what it shows (e.g., that EphA2 may be a promising target for new targeted therapies in TNBC based on preclinical laboratory findings) and doesn't show (e.g., EphA2 is a great target and clinical trials should start right away). Nitpicky? Maybe. But the burden is on the reporter to be clear and accurate. I'm being much kinder than scientific reviewers and grant reviewers who critique my work. Those folks regularly hand me my ass for much smaller offenses. We're a bunch of sticklers, *but we have to be.*

Our final mock article is really over the top, based on stuff I've actually read on the Internet on social media after conducting news searches. Fortunately, I don't often find this type of terrible reporting in legitimate news outlets. Other than inflated headlines from articles short on details, and, you guessed it, a lack of citations or links to the primary literature describing the study that was the subject of the report, reports from mainstream news outlets are generally fair and accurate. Even better, when I search Google for "breast cancer cure news" under the "news" tab from time to time, I find mostly legitimate news, which is always a relief. But every now and then, dubious articles from unreliable news sources show up in the mix and sometimes on the first page. I modeled this next example on one of those dubious articles. It has lots of red flags, starting with the headline.

"STUDY REVEALS BLOCKING A CELL-SURFACE RECEPTOR CURES BREAST CANCER EASILY" should immediately set off some major alarm bells. First off, "cure" is a buzzword that should always grab your inner skeptic's attention. And our study *doesn't* show that EphA2 cures breast cancer cells; it stops their growth, but the tumors are still hanging out in the laboratory animal and in the cell-culture dish. That's why the first mock article notes that future EphA2 inhibitors will likely be used with chemotherapy and other drugs in combination to *help kill* tumor cells more efficiently.

Moving on. Instead of giving a teaser with details of the study, the sentence below the headline reads, "Receptor stops cancer cells in their tracks." That doesn't inspire much confidence. The receptor *doesn't* stop cancer cells in their tracks. *Blocking* the receptor stops triple-negative breast cancer cell growth *in culture and in laboratory mice.*

The article might go on to report,

A new study provides a breakthrough for triple-negative breast cancer (TNBC), an aggressive form of breast cancer. TNBC cancer cells make too much EphA2, a cell-surface protein that makes cancer cells grow and spread. Right now, only toxic chemotherapy is used to treat TNBC, but this study provides hope for better therapies, including natural products found in plant extracts and green tea. What's the connection? Another study found that extracts and essential oils from plants like bearberry, Indian lilac, false black pepper, ginkgo biloba, giant crape myrtle, Indian gooseberry, pomegranate, bahera, and myrobalan block activity of EphA2 at nontoxic concentrations.[a]

Could these edible plants made by Mother Nature hold the key to keeping TNBC and other cancers at bay? Perhaps the science will lead us back to medicinal plants like ginkgo, lavender, and turmeric, used by ancient peoples, unlocking their secret health benefits.[b]

You can find extracts of these plants at retailers specializing in supplements.

a. Iftiin Hassan Mohamed et al., "Polyphenol Rich Botanicals Used as Food Supplements Interfere with EphA2-ephrinA1 System," *Pharmacological Research* 64, no. 5 (November 2011): 464–70, https://www.researchgate.net/publication/51479663_Polyphenol_rich_botanicals_used_as_food_supplements_interfere_with_EphA2-ephrinA1_system.

b. Shelby Deering, "Nature's 9 Most Powerful Medicinal Plants and the Science Behind Them: Chamomile," *Healthline*, updated February 28, 2019, https://www.healthline.com/health/most-powerful-medicinal-plants#chamomile.

So, using your newly acquired tools of investigation, what is wrong with this report? First, it neither includes a description of the study nor notes that the study was performed in animal models rather than in human clinical trials. The connotation of the word "toxic" for chemotherapy is negative and positive for the word "natural" in reference to plant-based medicines, which is misleading and points to a bias against standard-of-care therapy in favor of "alternative medicines" (as discussed in the previous chapter). Is chemotherapy toxic? Sure, but delivered in a medical setting in ways backed up by decades of research, it is effective.

The other article referenced[7] is legit and from a peer-reviewed journal, though the mock news article's link goes to a site that doesn't go directly to the open-access article. But this example of a bad news report took the study findings way out of context, failing to describe the rationale for looking at these plant extracts, the methods and chemistry, and the fact that the extracts blocked activity of EphA2 in cancer cell lines in a dish in the laboratory setting. There were no studies in laboratory animals looking at the pharmacokinetics in tumors after feeding the mice the plants or delivering the extracts in another way, no data on whether or not the active components within these extracts would last long enough in circulation to make it to tumors instead of

being cleared by the liver and/or kidneys. There were no toxicity studies. In other words, this study, like mine, is a preclinical laboratory
study. You'd have to look at the actual article and dig into the data to
realize all of this, since the news report didn't mention any of it.

If you only read this article, you might be tempted to go out and look
for supplements with these plant extracts. It's a little on the nose, since
the article even lets readers know they can find such supplements. It's
almost like it's an ad . . .

Also, beware of things allegedly used by "ancient people." Before the
era of modern medicine, you were as likely to die from bloodletting to
balance your "humors," mercury poisoning to treat your syphilis, or bacterial infections from cures made from animal shit.[8] "Ancient peoples"
didn't have the secret answers to health and wellness and didn't live
as long as modern humans who have access to antibiotics and other
modern medical interventions. The *Healthline* article related to the
medicinal value of plants and herbs that the reporter links isn't bad,
but the reporter of my mock piece doesn't include information about
safety and evidence for medicinal benefits included with the source.
That's also a red flag.

Again, this last mock article may seem a little over the top, but I
assure you that I based it on a real blog post I found that came up on a
search for news. And there are many more like it.

It is possible that the reporters who publish articles like this last
example are simply excited about particular studies and want to spread
the word—which is fine. What *isn't* fine, however, is publishing sensational, overblown headlines that can mislead readers into thinking that
"the cure" for cancer has, at last, been found. These are the kinds of
headlines that can get a lot of clicks and sell plenty of ads, but readers
would be served better with accuracy.

> *Bottom line:* when reading news reports about scientific studies,
> look for headlines that describe the nature of the study (e.g.,
> laboratory versus clinical or human trial) and present the find-
> ings without sensational claims. Look for a citation or link to
> the primary literature so you can review the study yourself, if you
> wish. Beware claims and statistics presented in the absence of
> source citations. Consider the source, and check the credibility
> of the newspaper, channel, blog, or other outlet reporting science

news. In my experience, articles like the last mock article tend to get passed along on social media outlets like Facebook, where clickbait is king and fact-checking is rare. Don't be fooled! Be a savvy news reader.

If you want to go one step further, check out PubPeer, an online database that fact checks published scientific manuscripts for mistakes, inaccuracies, and other poor reportage.[9]

After covering woo scams in the previous chapter and the variable quality of news coverage of science in this chapter, I'm going to shift gears and get personal in the next chapter. Becoming a breast cancer survivor changed me in many ways, including how I approach science and how I navigate not only the research aspects but the culture and politics of academia as well. As a woman, I'm not immune to sexism and the stereotypes and assumptions that come from sexism, and neither am I immune to gender-based harassment that the #MeToo movement has brought to light. The next chapter touches on these topics and how surviving cancer has given me the courage and conviction to own my career path and stand up for women in cancer research.

CHAPTER TWELVE

The Postcancer Feminist Manifesto

Academic-Researcher Edition

I've devoted a great deal of page space to the science of breast cancer. It seems only right that I spend a few pages on what scientists like me actually do and how many of us become academic researchers. Also, being a cancer patient and survivor has changed me in many ways, both as a scientist and as a human being. I'm not sure I'm the best example of an academic researcher—in fact, I've been called a great example of what *not* to do by more than a few senior scientists and colleagues. I only have one response to the doubters, the naysayers, and those scratching their heads, perplexed by the way I manage my life and career.

My response? *I'm still here.*

After twenty years (twenty-five if you count my years as a graduate student), I still get to spend a good bit of my time doing what I love—working at the laboratory bench, asking scientific questions, and experiencing the thrill of being the first person in the world to discover the answer with a new piece of data. The rest of my time is a slog through endless paperwork related to administrative, compliance, and financial laboratory-budget items (which I hate); preparing grant applications and scientific manuscripts (which I enjoy when my applications are funded and my manuscripts are accepted); mentoring students, postdoctoral fellows, technicians, and other laboratory staff (love); and sitting on committees like those that provide guidance for student thesis work (love) and those related to institutional operations and service (love/hate). At the end of the day, my favorite part of this job is the actual execution of laboratory science. I want to do the experiment. I want to see the results. I live for the challenges presented by unexpected and/or contradictory results, because that's where I find the most interesting answers, along with questions I hadn't even thought of yet.

It's the closest thing to magic I've ever experienced, and yet *it's science*. Logical, reproducible, testable science. My dear friend, fellow scientist and author A. J. Scudiere, once said, "Today's magic is tomorrow's science." She's right! And I get to live and work in that space. It is even more meaningful as a survivor. There are few things more cathartic than killing cancer cells in laboratory models whenever I get mad at breast cancer—which is often.

I'm still here, but my career path has been unconventional. When I entered my graduate program in 1995, the path for academic researchers was established, as was the accepted model of success.

Step one: Complete PhD training. This is a combination of

- classwork
- practical laboratory experience
- attending and giving seminars—in which you or someone else presents data from original research and receives feedback and inspires lively discussion (for the attendees who manage to stay awake)
- attending and giving lab-meeting presentations—in which you or someone else presents data from ongoing original research in progress and receives feedback and inspires lively discussion
- attending and giving journal-club presentations—in which someone presents a publication from the recent literature while the audience discusses its merits, picks it apart experiment by experiment, and trashes it while bragging/bitching about how they had that idea years ago and their own work is better
- attending scientific conferences and listening to leaders and up-and-comers in the field present their best original cutting-edge research (often while hungover [the attendees, not the speakers[1]])

- writing scientific manuscripts (badly) and revising them (extensively) until they're ready to submit for publication (after which they'll be trashed by peer reviewers whom you'll have to satisfy prior to acceptance)
- and writing grant proposals (badly) and revising them (extensively) until they're ready to submit for funding (see the bit about peer reviewers for scientific manuscripts).

Graduate school in biomedical research offers long hours, low pay—but at least we *get* paid, unlike many other grad students in nonscience fields—and the chance for advancement after passing qualifying exams designed to test your basic knowledge and critical-thinking skills, making sure you're ready to develop and execute a thesis project. A *note on the qualifying exams:* It was literally the hardest and most stressful exam I've ever endured, and it still gives me nightmares to this day. You learn how to formulate testable hypotheses, analyzing them using techniques you're learning as you go, screwing up, troubleshooting, screwing up again, and, on good days, finally getting them right and generating new, shiny, reproducible data that tells you whether your hypothesis is correct or whether you need to pursue a new, alternative hypothesis. You develop this into a cohesive thesis project that you complete in order to earn your degree.

When you've completed a thesis project and are ready to publish (or have published or are in the process of publishing at least one but preferably two or three papers), you write up your results in a thesis document that places your work in the broader context of the field and defend your thesis in a public presentation in front of your graduate mentor, a thesis committee, your fellow students, the postdoctoral fellows, your professors, your lab mates, your parents, and possibly your significant other. When your committee signs off on your thesis and you turn it in to the university and complete the requisite paperwork, you officially become a PhD—a doctor of philosophy—in your chosen field. Mine was cell biology.

Step two: Pack up and move to a different institution to complete postdoctoral training, which is much the same as graduate training, except you don't have to complete qualifying exams but you *do* have to apply for your own funding and work independently, which you've been trained to do. And if you haven't already done so as a graduate student, you begin to train students, technicians, and other junior post-doctoral fellows, developing the mentoring skills you'll need when you establish your own laboratory at yet another institution. It helps if you apply for and get career-development awards that support your transition to the coveted status of independent principal investigator—or a person who runs their own research program at a university or medical center.

Step three: Pack up and move to a different institution to establish your own laboratory as an assistant professor; get grants, recruit and train graduate students, postdoctoral fellows, and staff scientists; produce papers; find ways to serve the institution on various committees and in leadership roles; teach undergraduate and/or graduate courses; and travel to conferences and other institutions to present your work, garnering national and international recognition, creating a funding and publication portfolio worthy of the even more coveted status of associate professor, with tenure.

This may involve packing up and moving to a different institution one or more times.

So, how many times did *I* pack up and move? Zero. Zip. Zilch. None.

I graduated from my institution, accepted a postdoctoral training position at *gasp* *the same institution*, which, according to many (male) mentors in my circle, was a huge mistake—possible career suicide. Why? It comes from the traditional (male) model of career progression outlined above, harkening back to the days when academic institutes specialized in one area, so in order to expand your training and skill set you *had* to move. That wasn't the case when I was transitioning from graduate student to postdoc. The breadth and diversity of research directions, opportunities, and technologies available at my institution were and are enough to sustain near infinite training and growth opportunities.

But old ideas and notions die hard.

Did I kill my career by staying put? Obviously not, or I wouldn't be writing this book as an active academic researcher. When I accepted the postdoctoral position from my mentor, who later became a colleague and close friend, I was able to secure not one but two grants to support my training period, publishing around sixteen papers and building technical, writing, mentoring, and management skills that would carry me into the transition phase of my career after being promoted to research instructor and research assistant professor (nontenure track). I successfully applied for a career-development grant from the NIH. These grants are designed to support the transition to independence and to set trainees up to get their first major independent federal grant.

Thanks to that career-development grant, which covered my salary and research materials and supported some really incredible science, I was able to get my first independent-investigator grant, directing the research and working with some amazing research assistants and students and some phenomenal collaborators. Along the way, I met the love of my life, got married, and had a couple of kids. I had them during my postdoctoral training period, and juggling work with pregnancies and the pitiful six to eight weeks of paid maternity leave granted for each child while *not* falling behind and getting diverted onto the "Mommy Track" proved daunting.

This was the most stressful period of my life—even more stressful than enduring cancer, and that's saying something. But I stuck with it. And I'm still here. Isn't that success?

I've been thinking about this for a long time.

What does it take to be a successful working woman (in science)? Am I successful? Who defines success and the path to it (besides the tenure and promotions committee)? Why have I never wanted to do what half my graduate-level-course teachers told me I had to do in order to be successful? I really started thinking about it when I became a working mom. By the time I had my second child, figuring out what a successful working woman looks like had become kind of an obsession.

I think it's an obsession with women everywhere, regardless of what they do. Stay-at-home moms ask themselves if they're good enough and doing enough for their children. Working moms ask themselves if they're doing enough for their children *and* their outside jobs. Women without children (who are constantly pressured to have children) ask themselves if they're doing enough in their careers and in life. Women constantly question whether they're good enough—even Michelle Obama![2]

I think the answer boils down to following your own path and defining what success means to *you* rather than what you *think* it should mean based on the expectations of others. It took more than twenty years and enduring cancer for me to come to this conclusion, and it's been so liberating. At this point in my life and in my career, I'm no longer apologizing for who and what I am or how I do things. That was the birth of my manifesto. I encourage all women to make their own manifestos as a shield against self-doubt and as a source of empowerment. No matter who you are, what you do, or how you do it, *you are worthy*. You have value. You have so much to offer, and you do so much good in the world. Embrace that.

This is my working manifesto so far:

1. I will no longer apologize for my career path. Just because I haven't moved every seven years (zero desire to uproot and rebuild that often), haven't built a giant lab that I would have had to support by working eighty-hour weeks, and have interests and hobbies that don't revolve around science doesn't mean I am a loser or lack ambition or am a failure. I'm still working. I was funded before forty (meaning I got my first independent grant before the age of forty, which tells you how abysmal funding is). I'm proud of what I've accomplished. I am successful by the standards I've set for myself.

2. I will own what I love about the job—working at the bench, training students one on one at the bench (like the sorceress and her apprentices), making absolutely gorgeous data, and being the first person in the world to know something with each new result. It's awesome. This is why I became a scientist, and I will always make it a point to come back to the laboratory bench for the sheer joy of it.

3. I will acknowledge what I hate about the job and don't really want to do—schmoozing, trying to wrangle speaking engagements (though I finally learned to ask for help on that one), endless bureaucracy, and time-suck duties that take me away from the bench. I'll probably never love these aspects of the job, but I can reframe their value in my mind and embrace them as part of what allows me to do the parts of my job that I *do* love.

4. I will fight cancer in the lab and in my personal life on my own terms.

5. I will no longer apologize for being a working mom and for taking advantage of the flexibility that academic research can afford working parents. This is a biggie for me, because I spent way too many years avoiding conversations about my family life with (mostly male) colleagues for fear of being judged and dismissed. I refuse to do it any longer. My children are not a liability. My personal life isn't a liability. Motherhood isn't a badge of shame. It's a motherfucking badge of honor. I get more done in five to seven hours than many of my colleagues get done in eight to ten because I'm ruthlessly efficient, a master multitasker, a delegator, and a team player willing to trade my skill set and expertise with colleagues to get more shit done. My publication record proves it, no matter what that jackass reviewer for my last grant said.

6. I will stop hiding my work-life strategy and instead will celebrate and share it with colleagues, trainees, and my bosses, because I make this work and work well.

Would I have had the courage to embrace this manifesto before I had to face cancer? I don't know. But I do know that having cancer made me realize that a whole lot of worries and insecurities I'd harbored for years weren't worth my time. Cancer will show you what you're made of, and it will also teach you what's important. Ask anyone who has faced cancer, and they'll probably tell you that it narrowed their focus to what's truly important to them.

Toughening up and figuring out how to face cancer hasn't eliminated the challenges I still face today, but it's made me tougher and more determined to fight them. And though recent societal shifts haven't necessarily made it easier, these changes *have* taught me that I'm not alone. Many of the challenges I've faced as a woman in academia and as a woman in the patriarchy are shared by other women, and movements like #MeToo have helped us share our stories and shine a light on the burden women face due to the power imbalance that still persists due to gender inequality. Dr. Rita Colwell, with Sharon Berstch McGrayne, documents and discusses gender-based discrimination, sexism, and sexual harassment in her book *A Lab of One's Own: One Woman's Personal Journey Through Sexism and Science*.[3] From significant gaps in grant funding between male and female scientists to smaller laboratory spaces, salary gaps, and biases in hiring, sexism is, sadly, still very much alive and well in the sciences.[4]

All of the women in science I know have stories. Here are some of mine.

A few years ago, I confronted a male colleague who was berating female trainees in my laboratory for using the wrong hallway to transport laboratory animals. The area was under construction, and we believed the restrictions to have been lifted. I directed the trainees to take a different route and expressed my displeasure with the male colleague for speaking loudly and aggressively to them. As I walked back to my office, he followed me and proceeded to get into my personal space, speaking to me as if he were a schoolmaster scolding a naughty child, telling me that I "knew better" than to use that hallway and that he was going to report me and my staff for noncompliance. After asking him to take a step back and to speak to me in a normal, nonaggressive tone, I noted that I had directed my staff to use a different hallway and that if he didn't stop harassing me I would report him. He accused me of being aggressive (because I stood up for myself?) and told me I should watch my tone (projection and gaslighting much?).

We went back and forth, he said something rude, and then he walked away, leaving me leaning against my office door with a racing heart and a mind full of questions. This kind of thing had happened before, and more often than not I'd just shrugged it off and let it slide. I had been forced by the internalized misogynistic voices in my head (that need to STFU) and the external "well-meaning" voices around me to assess my *own* motives. *Should I have spoken up in defense of my female colleagues in the face of what was maybe no big deal? Did I overreact? Should I have backed down and deescalated the situation, apologizing for my audacity? Should I have been nicer?*

No.

No is a powerful word, isn't it? No, I wasn't looking for attention. I wasn't trying to make a scene. I wasn't the great Feminazi Crusader, out to get every male in my sphere. I was a supervisor who'd witnessed inappropriate behavior on the part of a colleague, the targets of which were three young, vibrant, female scientists who shouldn't have to put up with that kind of mistreatment. The cycle of silence is what allows this type of misbehavior to persist and gives tacit license to aggression and dominance on the part of men in the workplace because they are taught that they are entitled, *and they believe it.*

And why wouldn't they? No one ever tells them otherwise.

All of the times I hadn't spoken up flashed through my memory, as did the terror, the anger, the humiliation, and the regret that I'd said and done nothing.

I hadn't spoken up when I was fourteen years old and an older high school boy (whom I had a crush on) ripped my button-up denim skirt in a crowded hallway. *He gave me attention; it meant he liked me, right?* That's what I'd been taught. *You don't want to get him in trouble. You're the one who'll look bad, since you must have been flaunting your body to get his attention.* That's what I'd been taught. *Forget about it. Move on.*

But I didn't forget about it. I never wore that skirt again.

I didn't speak up when I was sixteen and working as a hostess at a local steak house. An old man came to my hostess station regularly to "say hello." He called me "Purty Legs," flashed wads of cash at me, and asked me if I'd like to go out with him so he could show me a good time. I was sixteen. He was at least sixty. *Forget about it. Move on. It's no big deal. Of course he wanted to take you out. I mean, come on, you do have nice legs, a big ass, and perky young breasts. It's not his fault he's attracted to you, a child, a virgin. It's natural.*

But I didn't forget, and I was always on my guard when he showed up during my shifts.

I didn't speak up when I was twenty-one, at a dance club where a group of men began dancing around me, grinding against my backside, leering. I giggled. I was terrified and didn't know what to do, trying my best to back away without offending them. *They were giving me attention, right? I should be flattered.* That's what I'd been taught. My amazing group of girlfriends took me by the arms and led me away. They were baffled. *Why did I let those men do that?* I didn't know what to say.

I did learn from it, though. Later, when a man at a bar put his hand on my knee and started squeezing, I pulled away and told him to stop. I got called a bitch for my trouble.

I didn't speak up as a graduate student when I was belittled or ignored by male faculty while male students got to engage. I didn't speak up when a male faculty member interviewing me said that I should join his institution's graduate program because there were a lot of young men there and I could find a husband. I didn't speak up during a career-counseling session when my male mentor asked if I planned to "get married and have a family." He didn't ask the male graduate students this; I know because I asked them. I didn't speak up when a powerhouse in the field advised me against marriage until I was thirty and asked me if I knew how to use birth control. I didn't even work for this jerk. He has four children. Obviously, *he* didn't know how to use birth control.

I've never forgotten that. He gave all of the women in his sphere of influence that same "sage advice." He probably still does. It's not legal. It's not right. But no one has taught him that, and if they tried, he'd probably retaliate.

I didn't speak up when I received a grant review that noted the number of publications I had produced under Brantley-Sieders, my "current last name." Yes, I have a hyphenated name. No, this reviewer didn't have to make an issue about it, but of course he did. I'm 95 percent certain the reviewer was male. My name has no bearing on my productivity or credentials. It just means that I'm a married woman who decided to compromise with my surname. The "current last name" note in the review was unnecessary, petty, and sexist.

No, I didn't get that grant. But I got the next one for which I applied. Success is my revenge.

This next one cuts deep.

I found out a male colleague and collaborator whom I deeply respected had advised one of his postdocs to pursue a career outside of academics. She was pregnant at the time and producing as much if not more data than her nonpregnant or male colleagues. He was supposed to know better. *Be* better. I still work with him, but I'll forever be guarded, keeping him at arm's length, and respecting him less.

Back to the most recent incident, where the colleague got in my face after I warned him off mistreating my female students. I hadn't wanted to have a confrontation with this man, and I hadn't wanted any trouble. But do you know what I really want? What *all* women want? We'd like to live in a world where we don't have to worry about male aggression when we're going about our daily lives. I'd love to live in a world where my male supervisors are allies, calling out their fellow men to do better, to be better, to be more inclusive, and, for the love of Pete, to stop being sleezy.

I want to live in a world where women aren't belittled or ignored but are engaged and mentored. I want to live in a world where women's career advice isn't focused on marriage and kids—or, alternatively, where those conversations also take place with men; you know, *future husbands and fathers*. I want to live in a world where boys don't show they "like" you by ripping your skirt in the high school hallway or where old men don't sexually harass children. I want to live in a world of equality. Can we make that happen?

I'm doing my part. When I talked with a female friend about this incident with my aggressive male colleague, she advised me to report it. "Look," she said, "you don't have to go all out and ask for an investigation if you don't want to, but here's the thing: If we don't report, it will keep happening. The older generation just put up with it, and if we keep putting up with it, our daughters will face the same challenges. Make a paper trail. If he does it again, the next victim will have more credibility[5] and a better chance of getting justice from the powers that be."

She was right. I reported the incident. I cc'd my supervisors, and I was supported. Both my longtime collaborator and mentor and my division chief, women for whom I have the deepest respect, stopped by my office to personally offer their support and to thank me for standing up for my colleagues. That's what we need to make a change. I'm part of the solution. I'm raising two children, one male and one female, to be part of the solution. I'm married to an ally who is part of the solution, looking out for his female colleagues in his own job and calling out his male colleagues when they step out of line.

I hope we can all be part of the solution.

Speaking of being part of the solution, in the next chapter I want to discuss how in the pursuit of science related to human disease we have become caught up in a trend that could do more harm than good. That trend, and its interpretation, deals with an emphasis on "exciting" science that "makes large leaps" rather than "incremental advances." Good in theory, but as I'll discuss in the next chapter, incremental advances are the backbone of science, and the quest for incorporating the newest technologies, the latest hot trend that everyone is chasing, and the most novel, exciting mechanisms shouldn't come at the expense of so-called "boring" science that has the potential to directly impact patients.

~

CHAPTER THIRTEEN

"Boring Science" and Why Chasing New and Shiny Isn't Always the Best Goal

I've been working in academic breast cancer research since 2000— 1997 if you count my graduate work—and I've seen peaks and valleys in funding, and hot new trends that have come and gone. I witnessed milestones, including the cloning and identification of specific mutations in BRCA genes, FDA approval of the first aromatase inhibitor and the HER2-targeted therapy trastuzumab, FDA approval of CDK4/6 inhibitor, the initiation of The Cancer Genome Atlas (TCGA, which curates data from tumor genomes and gene expression from thousands of human cancers), and the power of big data. We've made huge advances in the field that directly led to and continue to lead to better outcomes for patients—a fancy way of saying patients don't die as quickly and sometimes don't suffer as much. In the United States, breast cancer deaths have decreased 40 percent from the nineties through 2017 thanks to earlier detection and advances in treatments, including those mentioned above.[1] Quality of life issues notwithstanding—which are *huge* and which should be a bigger concern for clinicians and the research community—things are getting better for cancer patients in general and breast cancer patients in industrialized nations in particular.

These large leaps would not be possible without "boring science."

By "boring science"—a term I borrowed from a colleague on a recent study section but is by no means exclusive to him—I mean the kind of science that doesn't get peer reviewers excited. In today's parlance from requests *for* applications (RFAs) from federal and foundation funding sources, we should all be engaging in the kind of science that moves "from incremental advances to transformative innovation" and leads to "accelerated progress toward ending breast cancer" and "innovative research strategies."[2] Laudable goals, right?

Maybe, but incremental advances and tackling ongoing clinical problems using tools and knowledge that we already have—like molecular pathways we've already identified and studied (there aren't many new oncogene and tumor-suppressor pathways left to discover) and testing drugs we've already developed in new malignancies or in new combinations, the so-called "boring science"—have helped bring about clinical practices that have had a significant impact on patients, which is, or should be, the ultimate goal of what we do.

"Boring science" could mean conducting preclinical research using standard techniques to test for synergy and improved efficacy between two different FDA-approved drugs. In other words, slogging away in cell lines and animal models to test if the combination of two drugs does a better job than each drug alone by (1) improving the effectiveness of the treatment such that patients get a bigger benefit for longer, hopefully without horrible side effects, (2) preventing or overcoming drug resistance such that patients get a bigger benefit for longer, hopefully without horrible side effects, and/or (3) improving tumor killing and/or cutting down on the chances that the tumor will come back such that patients get a bigger benefit for longer, hopefully without horrible side effects.

If this sounds just as important or more important to you than chasing a new technique, finding a new drug target or strategy that could take more than a decade to make it to the clinic, or chasing the new hot trend in the field to get more funding because that's where the money is (e.g., "sexy" science like the proposed virus-cancer connection in the '70s and '80s, angiogenesis inhibitors in the '80s and '90s, tyrosine kinase inhibitors in the '90s and 2000s, tumor metabolism and harnessing antitumor immunity in 2010 and beyond), then you might be surprised and dismayed to know that leadership and peer reviewers in funding agencies do *not* seem to agree. The idea of the next big thing isn't unique to cancer research or science in general. Those types of discoveries get you high-profile papers in high-impact journals, they get peer reviewers and study sections excited, they build and sustain careers; but do they ultimately benefit patients?

Not necessarily.

In terms of the examples of "sexy science" across various decades discussed above, the benefit to patients has been a bit of a mixed bag. Turns out, very few human cancers are induced by viruses (cervical cancer is one notable exception).[3] In spite of buzz and promising preclinical data surrounding antiangiogenic agents, "wonder drugs" in this category, angiostatin and endostatin never made it to the clinic, and anti-VEGF drugs failed to live up to the hype surrounding them.[4] On the other hand, tyrosine kinase inhibitors have been a game changer for cancer treatment (see more on this back in chapter 5), and harnessing antitumor immunity has produced phenomenal results in select malignancies and patients (see chapter 16). The problem is, there's no way to predict which trend in scientific research will yield more effective treatment options for cancer. On the other hand, the decades of "boring," basic science work that identified and characterized the genes included in tumor gene-expression-profiling tests like Oncotype DX and MammaPrint (see chapter 4) have revolutionized patient outcomes by predicting recurrence risk and sparing patients who will not benefit from chemotherapy the hell of enduring chemo.

That doesn't mean we shouldn't push for innovation, but we have to balance that with risk, reward, and the everyday "boring" studies that lead to major advances. From "boring" investigation of bacterial genetics that led to advances like CRISPR/Cas9 gene editing, "boring" analysis of soil samples from a remote island that led to the discovery of rapamycin and a host of new molecularly targeted therapies used to treat breast and other cancers,[5] and "boring" studies of worm genetics that led RNA-interference technology and the discovery of microRNA, the significance of each of these initial studies could not have been anticipated at the time of initial funding and support, but think what might have happened had we *not* cast our funding and scientific-support net wide.

Here's an example that's a bit closer to home for me. I'll call it "A Tale of Two Projects." At the time of this writing, I am an assistant professor of medicine, tenure track, currently supported by two multi-PI federal research grants (not much), funding for an insanely talented medical student for one year of laboratory research, and what's left of the start-up package I received in 2015 and later in 2021. I have a gap in my publication record for 2018 due to time off for my own personal cancer battle—which has been held against me in a recent grant application—and I desperately need money for research. I have two projects in mind for my next grant application. I'll probably submit both as applications, but I'm fairly certain which one is more likely to be funded. *Note:* Both projects are good, quality science. I'm not knocking either. I'm just making a point about the current trends in funding and how they sometimes favor new and shiny at the expense of standard yet translatable.

Project 1. Determine if combination therapy targeting EphA2 receptor tyrosine kinase and CDK2/4 inhibitors synergize in basal-like, triple-negative breast cancer (see chapter 11 for information on EphA2 and cell cycle, which is what CDK2/4 inhibitors target).

Don't get hung up on "EphA2" and "CDK2/4." Just think of them as two drug targets with two drugs. With me so far? I hope so. Drug 1 (targets EphA2) isn't FDA approved, but a new therapeutic is showing promise in Phase I/II clinical trials. Drug 2 (targeting CDKs including CDK2) is close to FDA approval. We know a *lot* about how drug targets 1 and 2 make cells grow, help them move, and keep them alive in cancer. That makes them, from a funding and peer-review perspective, "boring."

Seriously, we've reached a state in cancer research where knowing a lot about molecules and pathways makes them less "novel," not as exciting without some new technological or mechanistic spin, and not as fundable. The question of whether or not the research is likely to help patients in the clinic seems less important than novelty.

We also know a bit about what EphA2 and CDK2/4 do in basal-like, triple-negative breast cancer—a type of cancer that, while only representing relatively few breast cancer diagnoses, hits younger women, disproportionally affects women of African descent, and is super aggressive and lethal. Until recently, nothing was available to these patients except chemotherapy, and there is only one currently approved molecularly targeted therapy (sacituzumab govitecan; see chapter 5). I'm going to propose testing the effect of these two drugs in cell lines, in mice with tumors (lots of different complementary models), and I'll probably throw in some studies pairing them with chemotherapy (because everyone with this type of cancer gets chemo) and with immune-checkpoint inhibitors (hot topic right now, relevant for this type of breast cancer, and if the combo makes tumors responsive to antitumor immunity, that would be *great*). While we might not find anything new and exciting in terms of biology, there's a decent chance that we'll find a combination that may improve drug effectiveness and could be translated to the clinic.

Project 2. Determine if modified siRNAs that use serum albumin as an endogenous nanocarrier can effectively target conventionally undruggable drivers of basal-like, triple-negative breast cancer.

Don't get hung up on the lingo with "siRNA" and "serum albumin" and "nanocarrier." Basically, my (amazing) collaborators and I want to use a strategy that will allow a gene-therapy agent, siRNA—which targets mRNA-encoding cancer drivers for destruction, thereby preventing translation to protein—to hide in the bloodstream by latching on to stuff that's already in blood, reach tumor cells, enter the tumor cells, and kill them. Nanotechnology is still relatively new, and while lots of carriers are being developed, few are used in the clinic.

This is exciting, novel, and decidedly not "boring"—though we've still been dinged by peer reviewers because the *idea* of using serum albumin as a carrier isn't new. *Sighhhhh . . .*

In spite of the novelty and excitement, there are a ton of things that could go wrong and that could derail the whole approach: the siRNA might get shredded by blood flow, cleared by the liver or kidneys, or eaten up by immune cells looking for stuff that doesn't belong in the body; the siRNA might not get into the tumor, or it may only hit the cells that are easiest to reach; the siRNA might not get to the right place in the cell and might get chewed up by the cell's garbage disposal (lysosome). Our initial studies suggest these things won't happen, but you never know. We could find out all kinds of cool and exciting things about how nanocarriers affect physiology and interact with tumor cells in living animals. We can image the process, making really cool pictures that reviewers like in papers and grant applications. We could discover a lot of really cool things about the biology. While we may provide a stepping-stone to clinical relevance, that will likely take more than a decade—but probably longer, since it's "proof-of-concept" science and the nanocarriers will have to be refined, redesigned, and tested a lot before then.

Project 1 is "boring" science that may have a better chance of helping patients more quickly. Project 2 is exciting science that is "innovative" and "more than incremental" in terms of advance and is just so freakin' cool! I'm excited about both projects and would love to get funding for each of them. Which is the better project? That likely depends on whether or not you are looking at it from a scientist's perspective or a patient's perspective. Project 2 may be more likely to generate exciting, high-impact papers, may be more likely get more attention and more opportunities for speaking engagements and networking, and is more likely to advance my career. Project 1 may be more likely to help patients sooner but probably won't yield high-impact papers or get a lot of national attention (until and unless it goes to the clinic, and then it will be the folks running the trials who get all of the "glory"). Of course, some of the reception depends on how I spin and sell the research; the grantsmanship part is on me. The fact that I'm a survivor might help with study sections that include patient advocates. But I think it's fair to predict that project 2 is what I need to advance my career.

I want to do both projects, actually, but my heart and hope is with project 1. I want to make a difference to patients. It would be nice to be able to do that in my lifetime. I've spent the past two decades working on one of the drug targets in project 1, watching a drug go to clinical trials only to be ditched when the company that made the drug was bought by a larger company and the project and trial were nixed. As of March 8, 2021, there were 129 published papers supporting EphA2 as a driver of breast cancer progression. Ten of them are mine. The most recent provides evidence for EphA2 as a regulator for breast-to-bone metastasis,[6] and, if approved, new EphA2 inhibitors could be tested on metastatic breast cancer.

I really want this.

But I'm probably not going to get funded for project 1 unless I can come up with some novel angle or technology, and even then it might not be enough; recent reviews of my EphA2-based grants support this discouraging outlook. That sucks. I don't know how to change it, unless we as scientists and leaders who hold the purse strings make these types of studies a bigger priority. Or unless they're sponsored by pharma, which has a myriad of pros and cons and potential conflicts of interests that I won't discuss in the interest of time, focus, and minimal experience working with drug companies. In the coming years, however, I will continue to champion the "boring" science that is likely to lead to better outcomes for patients—as a peer reviewer for manuscripts and grant applications, in my capacity as an academic investigator, and as a patient advocate. "Boring" science matters.

And I'm going to keep submitting grants until I get funding for project 1 in some form or another. I'm more encouraged based on reviews from a recent submission to a foundation that specializes in providing seed money to support projects of merit that will likely be federally funded if investigators can generate preliminary data. And project 2 is likely to get funded after a much-needed increase in the NCI payline[7] and after five previous submissions. I'm grateful to have ongoing research funding support and time.

I'm determined to get this done.

Next up, we're going to move into the final portion of the book that focuses on breast cancer survivorship and finding a new normal. I'll cover managing the long-term, chronic aspects of breast cancer, sexual health and getting your groove back as a breast cancer survivor, and moving forward with humor and hope. This section will include information about some really exciting advances in breast cancer research and treatment, like antitumor immunity and breast cancer vaccines.

I truly believe that things are getting better for breast cancer patients and survivors and that things will continue to improve.

PART IV

~

SURVIVORSHIP AND
FINDING A NEW NORMAL

CHAPTER FOURTEEN

~

My Condition Is Chronic, but My Tits Are Iconic

One thing I've learned about cancer after my diagnosis is that cancer is a long-term condition. I'll be taking estrogen blockers for ten years total. The almost three years I've been taking them have changed my body and wreaked havoc on my sex life. (More on that later, along with some tools that have helped.) These medications are also wreaking havoc on my liver, something I'm working on with my oncologist and primary-care provider to manage and correct. It will require some lifestyle changes and possibly a medication switch, and I suspect I'll continue to face issues like liver damage, bone loss, and other side effects for at least the next seven years.

Since we found residual disease after my first surgery, I'm still in the process of breast reconstruction, three years after my initial diagnosis. I've completed one revision after my autologous DUG flap procedure in order to better match the left reconstructed breast to the right intact breast, and I'll likely need at least two more revisions (see chapter 16 for progression photos). Multiple surgeries have affected my body and my mental health, and I worry about the long-term impacts on my general health. Fatigue is an ongoing issue for me, and I worry it's becoming chronic.

I didn't realize that this was a possibility when I was first diagnosed. I thought I'd have surgery, then I'd get a course of radiation and take my medications, and, aside from a few manageable side effects, I'd go on with life as usual.

Yeah, I was that naive.

According to the CDC's National Center for Chronic Disease Prevention and Health Promotion, cancer is actually one of seven chronic diseases affecting six in ten adults in the United States, with four in ten having two or more chronic diseases. The other chronic diseases listed include heart disease, chronic lung disease, stroke, Alzheimer's disease, diabetes, and chronic kidney disease,[1] but there are more. Autoimmune conditions like rheumatoid arthritis, fibromyalgia, Hashimoto's autoimmune thyroiditis, celiac disease, and Graves' disease are chronic, as are depression and generalized anxiety disorder. Read Jenny Lawson— aka the Bloggess, aka one of the funniest people on the planet and champion of misfits everywhere—for more on chronic anxiety, depression, and rheumatoid arthritis.[2] Her candid descriptions of what it's like to live with these conditions and how she copes are funny as hell and inspiring.[3] She was a big influence for me and helped inspire this book.

These diseases and conditions are as unique as the patients who deal with them, but they do have a few elements in common. For example, unlike acute illnesses, where you feel terrible but know it will end after a short period of time, chronic illnesses have no time limit for misery; that's why they're chronic. In addition to the symptoms of the chronic illness or disease itself, you have to deal with the stress and anxiety related to managing the chronic illness.[4] Stressors like uncertainty about the future and how unpredictable the disease itself can be, worries about disability or frustration with days when your chronic illness prevents you from completing tasks or doing the things you love, and the financial stress that comes from difficulties working and the expense of treatments can all add up and compound the negative effects on your health and well-being.[5]

I worry about how fatigue is affecting my work in the lab. Some days I'm full of energy and can juggle multiple experiments, manage and mentor students and staff, come home and help with homework and dinner prep, and still have energy to do yard work and other household chores. Other days I'm so tired I need to take multiple naps and find getting up to feed myself a Herculean task. That's chronic illness. It's sneaky. It doesn't care about your plans or goals or schedule. Some days

I can function with minimal aches or pain from healing surgical incisions and medication side effects. Some days I need a lot of over-the-counter pain meds, but then I worry about how this extra medication on top of all the other meds I take are going to affect my liver.

It truly feels like I'm damned if I do, damned if I don't.

I look at my body, which is still very much a work in progress, and wonder if I'll ever get used to these new breasts that don't feel like they belong to me. Is the quest for symmetry and having a pair of matching tits worth the stress and pain of more surgery? My current cycle is to recover, get back on my feet and get back to the lab on a regular (COVID-permitting) schedule for weeks or a few months, then have more surgery that puts me back in recovery mode. It's irrational, but I feel like just when I'm getting back to normal and moving on with my life, cancer reminds me that it's still in charge.

Cancer is a shitty boss. I'm ready to quit working for it and around it.

So, what can *you* do manage breast cancer as a chronic condition? First off, I recommend seeking support from mental health-care professionals as well as from other patients and survivors (see more on this in chapter 8). There's something about knowing you're not alone and sharing experiences—triumphs, setbacks, frustrations, successes, and everything that comes with being in the survivor club—that's so comforting. Next, I recommend giving yourself a break and permission to listen to your body and follow its lead as much as possible. On bad days when I'm filled with fatigue, I give myself permission to sit down and rest. If I can squeeze in a power nap, I take it, even if that means I have to adjust my expectations for what I can accomplish that day. That was so tough for me to learn to do, since I live by to-do lists and derive a great deal of satisfaction from ticking off items I've finished. When I have items that I haven't finished, I feel terrible—like I'm not doing enough or trying hard enough. Circling back to mental-health resources and tools, reframing my thoughts to avoid catastrophizing (indulging in *I'm so far behind I'll never catch up* kind of thinking), mental filtering (focusing on what I haven't done instead of what I have accomplished), and banishing those terrible "should" statements (e.g., *I should be able to get all of this work done, because otherwise cancer wins*) gives me the weapons I need to be kind to myself and to focus on the positive.[6]

Note: I'm not talking here about embracing toxic positivity, which I'll cover in the next chapter. It's okay and *normal* to experience negative thoughts and to be afraid, to be sad, to be angry, and to acknowledge that cancer sucks. It's okay to *not* be okay. What I mean by focusing on the positive is reflecting on the very real good things in your life, work, and experiences. You have to grieve for what you've lost before you can accept what you have left when it comes to cancer and chronic conditions. Don't bury the pain, frustration, anger, and resentment and all of the other natural negative emotions and thoughts that you experience after diagnosis, as you go through treatments, and as you find your new normal. But process them in a healthy way.

One of the most common yet least researched and talked about side effects of cancer in general and breast cancer in particular is sexual dysfunction. This is a significant quality of life issue that often gets buried under "more pressing" matters like treatments to keep you alive. But it's a problem I've personally experienced, and I'm not alone. That's the bad news. The good news? There's actually something you can do about it. (More on some of the current interventions available below.) Please, please, *please* talk to your health-care team about this issue. It's nothing to be ashamed of; maintaining a healthy sex life (if you're into sex—there's no shame if you are and no shame if you're not) is an important part of overall health and well-being.

Sex and Breast Cancer: Getting Your Groove Back

Breast cancer can wreak havoc on a woman's body image along with a woman's body. Coupled with some of the nastier side effects that come with cancer therapies like chemotherapy and especially estrogen blockers—including vaginal dryness, loss of sexual desire and/or the ability to respond, and loss of sensation—breast cancer can have a terrible effect on your sex life. Women are already at a disadvantage in terms of research and a fundamental understanding of the complexities of female sexual responses relative to dudes. Sadly, there are many forces in society and the health-care industry that trivialize the impact of the sexual side effects of cancer therapy on a patient's quality of life. If you're like me, you've heard one or more of the following bullshit statements when you've complained to friends, family, or some health-care providers: "The focus is to keep you alive and keep the cancer at bay, right? Sex should be the least of your worries." "That stuff goes away as you get older anyway." Or my personal least favorite that makes me stabby: "There are other forms of intimacy, like cuddling or hand-holding, and you can still satisfy your husband."

I read that last one online, and I'm 99.99 percent certain a man came up with it.

I call bullshit, and you should, too. Sexual satisfaction is an essential part of life and health for *all* humans who are into sex (again, no shame if you're asexual and it's not your thing), including women. It infuriates me that there are three FDA-approved boner pills on the market for men (Viagra, Cialis, Levitra) but *no* equivalent arousal aid for women. When I asked my former gynecologist about issues with waning sensation in my clitoris and problems reaching climax, she shrugged and told me about all she could do was prescribe testosterone cream.

I tried it. It didn't work for me. That's not to say it won't work for you, but (1) talk to your oncologist about the risk of topical testosterone absorption and aromatization to estrogen if you have ER+ breast cancer, and (2) there *are* other options. My former gyno was either misinformed or less concerned with her cancer and postmenopausal patients that she was about her pregnant patients. Are there enough treatment options out there for female sexual dysfunction? Definitely not. But after a frank conversation with my medical oncologist that, while awkward, was necessary and handled with sensitivity and professionalism (by my medical oncologist; I giggle snorted my way through it), I got a referral to the Women's Institute for Sexual Health (WISH) clinic.[7]

It was enlightening and game changing!

Thanks to the amazing health-care providers at WISH, I was introduced to Revaree, a hyaluronic acid–based vaginal moisturizer that helps maintain lubrication and heal thinning vaginal skin.[8] This one has personally helped me build an oasis out of the dry desert my poor vajazzle had become. It's pricey and not covered by insurance, which are downsides. Avoid using Vaseline, as well as olive and coconut oils. The former can put you at risk for yeast infections, and the oils can irritate your vagina or cause allergic reaction. There are other vaginal moisturizers on the market, and, like lube, they can really help ensure penetrative sex is comfortable and *not* painful.

Sex shouldn't be painful, and if it is, you shouldn't be expected to grin and bear it. And just so we're clear, *of course* sex isn't limited to penetrative sex. Whatever excites and arouses you, gets you off, and satisfies your desires for pleasure and intimacy is sex. That was true for your precancer body, and it's still true for your postcancer body. One of the best things you can do to love your postcancer body and to find what feels good is to explore on your own. Hopefully you discovered what feels good with your body during puberty, so think of this new phase as a voyage of rediscovery. Even if you have a partner, you might be more comfortable starting on your own. Breast sensation changes after surgery, even lumpectomy. Be patient with your tender skin as it heals and as nerve endings come back online. Even after it heals, the psychological impact of enduring a cancer diagnosis and treatment can make your body feel foreign, like a wounded animal that needs protection, or like your enemy. These feelings and emotions are normal. I'm a big proponent of therapy, and we've covered taking care of mental, emotional, and spiritual health (chapter 8). Taking care of mental health will help the other aspects of health and acceptance of your new body. But in the meantime, try and make peace with your body and see it as your ally. It has carried and nurtured you throughout your life, and you've battled cancer together.

Love your body like the warrior it is.

Sexual arousal and sensation are a bit tougher to tackle than vaginal dryness, but I'll share some other recommendations and advice I received from the WISH clinic. The company Bonafide, maker of Revaree, also sells a product called Ristela, which is marketed to help with arousal and sexual response.[9] It's an injectable, which isn't ideal, but it reportedly works wonders with some women. I can't recommend this product one way or another, but I'm including any and all available safe tools in the arsenal to help cancer patients find their "O" faces.

If you haven't ever tried toys, treat yourself! And even if you have, there are so many new options on the market that can get you revved up. Focus on toys that stimulate the clitoris, which is the best bet for a ticket to Climax Town. Toys that penetrate the vagina are also beneficial in fighting off vaginal atrophy—also called *atrophic vaginitis*, a condition caused by reduced estrogen, causing inflammation, dryness, and thinning of vaginal walls.[10] Risk factors for developing vaginal atrophy include loss of ovarian function (menopause or medically induced menopause after chemotherapy or radiation) and use of SERMs like tamoxifen and AIs like letrozole. Smoking poses an additional risk. Even worse, sexual effects are often accompanied by urinary problems, like frequent urination, urinary tract infections, burning or pain during urination, and stress incontinence (e.g., peeing a little when you laugh, sneeze, cough, jump, or run). While hormone replacement therapy is a no-go for ER+ breast cancer patients (for which estrogen makes cancer cells grow), moisturizers, lubricants, and stretching with intercourse and/or dilators are all possibilities for improving sexual function. If you experience pain during intercourse, your health-care team or gynecologist may recommend dilation with increasingly larger dilators over time. A relatively new drug that falls into the SERM class, ospemifene (trade names Osphena and Senshio), is approved for treatment of dyspareunia (pain during intercourse), which plagues breast cancer patients and survivors suffering from vaginal atrophy.

Another option is vaginal laser treatment (aka *vaginal rejuvenation*[11]). It sounds scary, I know. (A laser to the lady bits??) But what it actually does is stimulate fibroblast cells in the urogenital tract to produce more collagen and also increase natural lubrication and pH balance. The two laser types are carbon dioxide microablative laser therapy and Erbium YAG nonablative photothermal laser therapy. These interventions are expensive and, sadly, not covered by insurance, but hopefully lobbying the health-care industry and lawmakers to pay more attention to female sexual health and interventions will change that. Write your congressional representatives,[12] and ask them to support funding for research on female sexual dysfunction through the National Institutes of Health. You can also support the American Association of Sexuality Educators, Counselors and Therapists and their advocacy work in the arena of sexual health.[13]

Having conversations with your health-care team about sexual dysfunction and sexual side effects can be challenging, especially for women for whom sex (or the pursuit of sexual pleasure) comes with the stigma of shame. When this is compounded by the lack of attention to female sexual health and function in the medical community—not to mention in society as a whole—many women suffer in silence, and that's the real shame. My advice? Start a conversation with your health-care team about sexual concerns. If your medical oncologist isn't receptive, ask for a referral to a urologist specializing in female urogenital conditions, or consider seeking care from another provider. If that isn't possible, talk to your gynecologist.

Also, if you have a partner, keep that person in the loop, and be honest about your struggles. Hopefully you have a supportive partner who is—and should be—patient, kind, and willing to experiment and explore new ways to bring you sexual pleasure. Experimenting and exploring are half the fun! Warm up with a toy, hopefully bringing you at least one orgasm, and then experiment with new positions and extended oral. Or give anal a try (go *slowly* with anal, and make sure you do the prep work with plugs, stretching, and *lots* of lube); it can be intimidating at first, but if you're missing vaginal and clitoral sensation, the incredible fullness and newness of backdoor sex (not to mention titillation from what is taboo for many women—gay guys have all the fun) can give a much-needed boost to your sex life. And, of course, there are plenty of racy romance novels, film and television devoted to the female gaze (*Dirty Dancing* and *Outlander* are two of my personal favorites) and sensual songs that can help put you in the mood and rev your engine.

No matter what you try, don't put too much pressure on yourself. Mental pressure is distracting and never good when you're going for an orgasm. Relax. Give whatever new avenue you explore a few tries, and then move on to something new. Communicate, communicate, communicate with your partner about everything from pain to body insecurities and fears, and, most especially, be clear about what feels good to you. Your partner isn't a mind reader. Tell them what's working. And don't give up. Remember, *you are worth it.*

And remember that you are also worthy of care, compassion, and support. In the next chapter, I'll discuss supports you can ask for—or provide for a friend or loved one who is diagnosed with cancer. I'll also cover what *not* to say and do, as well as the difference between support and toxic positivity.

CHAPTER FIFTEEN

~

The Top Ten Things You Can Say or Do When a Friend or Loved One Is Going Through Cancer, and What You Should Never Say or Do

When a friend or a loved one is facing cancer, it can be really tough to know what to say or do. Many people are afraid to bring up the subject because they think it will upset the person diagnosed. Others don't want to interfere with what they might perceive to be a private health matter. Many are afraid they'll say the wrong thing. Cancer is hard to talk about when it affects someone you love.

Then there are those self-appointed experts who know someone who went through cancer and want to tell you all the gory details, or they want to tell you to take this supplement or try that superfood even though they don't have personal experience with cancer or a medical degree; this type of person is very irritating. So are the Debbie Downers who have some sort of weird fascination with what terrible fate might await you with your cancer treatments, especially if they don't work. On the flip side, Pollyanna, the queen of positivity, won't let anything get her down and, by extension, won't allow *you* to be down, because *we just have to stay positive and happy all the time.* Then you have the people who want to pray for you, with you, or over you (that one's just so weird to me), the people who will tell you that you'll *absolutely* live or that you're *totally* going to die, and the trolls from the stinky bowels of the Internet who actually *hope* you die.

Obviously, these people embody how not to treat a person with cancer, even though some of them are well meaning. I've made a list of things you shouldn't say or do when someone you know is going through cancer. If you're worn out and tired of telling these people not to say or do stupid and/or insensitive stuff, feel free to simply hand them a copy of this list. Then you can go about your day without wasting precious time or oxygen when you should be focused on recovering.

The Top Ten Things You Should Never Say or Do When a Friend or Loved One Is Going Through Cancer (And What You Can Do Instead)

I have my own list with some items that are specific for me, but there's a lot of overlap with other published lists out there.[1] I'll cover what's wrong in each case and provide alternatives for support—which is important. There are some people you don't want to cut out of your life just because they mess up, but you also don't want them to keep messing up. I hope this helps.

Okay. What *not* to say:

1. These things happen for a reason.
2. At least you got the "good" kind of cancer.
3. Have you tried [insert supplement, diet, or other woo-woo thing]?
4. You must have done something to get it./What do you think caused your cancer?
5. I know someone who died from [breast] cancer.
6. You're lucky; some people have it way worse.
7. Oh no—I've always been terrified that I would get cancer!
8. Stay positive!
9. You're so strong/brave. You've got this!
10. God never gives you more than you can handle.

Let's unpack these, starting with #1.

Telling someone with cancer that "these things happen for a reason" is infuriating. No, these "things"—meaning *cancer*—happen because of random mutations and genetic changes in cells that make them go rogue. Can other external factors contribute to cancer? Sure. But speculating on what may have caused the cancer (without any evidence or likely any way of knowing what did) isn't helpful. (More on that with #4.) I also hate being told that I got cancer so I could be "an inspiration" for others or "find my purpose and calling." That's bullshit. Being told you're someone else's inspiration porn isn't helpful, and most of us already had a purpose or calling we were working on before cancer derailed us, thank you very much. Now, if the patient or survivor says they feel compelled or called to do outreach or activities to help other patients or survivors, that's their prerogative. But you don't get to say that to them or place them in that role.

Remember Patton Oswalt: It's chaos. Be kind.

Instead, try saying, "I'm so sorry this is happening to you."

On to #2, one of my least favorites and a statement that never fails to make me stabby. I've been told by regular folks and other survivors how lucky I am that I got the "good" kind of breast cancer or, worse, "baby" breast cancer. *Newsflash:* there's no such thing as "good" cancer or "baby" cancer.

It's cancer, and it sucks. Period.

I can sort of see where this one comes from. Regular people who are looking to be positive (in a misguided, fucked-up kind of way) may say this with the best of intentions, like as a way to cheer up the person with cancer. But it really doesn't cheer up the person with cancer. First of all, it minimizes their experience and makes them feel as if their pain and suffering don't matter. Second, saying this can add to the guilt they may already be experiencing. When I heard this from some friends, family, and people I trusted, it made me feel guilty for complaining about my situation because *I didn't need chemo, I had early-stage disease, and though I was hurting, stressed, and scared because of my cancer, I didn't have the right to be, right?*

That's the kind of toxic thinking that statements about "good" cancer can inspire. (More on that with #6.)

Hearing statements about "good" cancer and "baby" cancer from other survivors can be even worse. These people are your tribe; they're in the same exclusive club, and at their best they're your support system, your lifeline, and the people who truly understand what you're going through. They have your back. But sometimes when trading cancer

stories, comparisons bring up some negative emotions and those terrible "Why me?" questions that can lead to bitterness and lashing out.

"Oh, this person was diagnosed with breast cancer at stage I? That's
just baby cancer. I had stage III."

"You think *you* had it bad, *I* had radiation *and* chemo!"

"Whatever—I have stage IV. Y'all have nothing on me."

I would argue that it's perfectly valid for a person with cancer to
have these thoughts and feelings; all thoughts and feelings are valid.
Don't bury the feelings; *process* them. But this doesn't mean that you
have to voice those thoughts and feelings to diminish someone else's
situation. It's not a contest; it's cancer, and it sucks for every person
who gets diagnosed. Talk to loved ones or a therapist, rail at the universe—do what you need to get through, but don't take it out on your
fellow survivors.

Be kind.

As we've talked about in previous chapters, woo-woo "treatments"
for cancer don't work, and they can even be harmful. So as for #3,
those well-meaning suggestions about trying this diet, that vitamin, a
series of essential oils, or other nonmedically tested or recommended
"treatments" is super problematic. If you're tempted to give this advice
to someone who has cancer, *just don't*. They've already had several
conversations with their health-care team, they've scoured the Internet, they're trying to get through treatments with their bodies and
sanity intact, and they don't need a lecture on the merits of a vegan/
gluten-free/plant-based/no-sugar/free-range/paleo diet or whatever diet
is currently trending. Seriously, if someone facing cancer wants to eat
a cheeseburger (especially after surgery or completing chemo), *let them
eat their fucking cheeseburger in peace*. It's like talking to someone about
their weight: If they don't ask for or invite your opinion, just don't.
Don't say it.

"But my cousin swears by antioxidants!"

Don't.

"Weed cured my uncle's cancer."

No, it fucking didn't. Just don't.

"If you do intermittent fasting and low carb, you'll be cancer free!"

No specific diet will guarantee that you'll be cancer free. Just don't.

Look. Eating healthily and exercising, being tobacco free, not drinking to excess, and embracing other healthy lifestyle habits are definitely recommended by health-care providers. None of these lifestyle choices will hurt you, and they can all improve your overall health. But none of them is a sure-fire way to stay cancer free. They can certainly reduce your risk, but you may still get cancer. You didn't get cancer because you smoked a few cigarettes in college or ate junk food through most of your twenties. You didn't get it because you have a glass of wine every now and again or because you skipped cardio day at the gym a few days (or weeks, or months, or years). You may still get cancer no matter your lifestyle and personal choices. It's chaos. Be kind.

This also relates to #4—"You must have done something to get it./ What do you think caused your cancer?" Whenever someone asks me what I think caused my cancer, I'm tempted to lean in really close and loud whisper, "*I think it was you.*" Mean? Maybe, but it's such a stupid question. What I *really* think is that I had crap luck in the genetic/ DNA-repair cycle in my boobs, and, *boom*—cancer. But that's not what they're really asking. No, many of them will bring up things like lifestyle or weight.

I'm fat. No bones about it, just lots of adipose. I've struggled with my weight for most of my adult life, and I've dealt with body-image issues created by our society's ridiculous beauty standards for women (that somehow don't extend to men). Fortunately, I've learned to love and accept my body and to be content as a curvy size fourteen woman with a juicy booty—though much smaller tits. I'm much more concerned about health than the number on the scale, but given the link between obesity and breast cancer risk, the assumption these people are making with their concern trolling is implied.

What they really mean is *Oh, you're fat; that's probably why you got breast cancer.*

But is that true? Did my weight contribute to the malignant transformation of my cells that led to breast cancer? Maybe, but there are so many factors involved in cancer besides body mass and metabolism that I'll never know for sure. Is it super shitty to ask someone who's had cancer if they think they got it because they're too fat? That's easy. It *is* super shitty, so don't ask.

It's more than okay to wonder about what causes cancer. I've spent my entire career trying to unlock the molecular processes that turn normal cells into malignant cells and how to stop it. But asking a person with cancer what they think *caused* their cancer is such a loaded question that has no good answers and can lead to a whole lot of guilt-fueled thoughts about what they may have done to put themselves at risk. No one deserves cancer; it's not a punishment from the universe, karma, or some divine entity. It's chaos. Be kind. Don't ask stupid, insensitive questions.

Also, to quote Jon Stewart, one of the funniest people to ever grace my television screen, "When in doubt, don't be douchey."[2]

This next one, #5, really chaps my ass. It's so very unhelpful. Telling someone who has cancer about the people you know who've died from the disease serves no purpose, is awkward as hell, and is just really not the kind of thing you say. We all know people who've died from cancer. It's a terrible disease that can and does steal lives; but no one who has been diagnosed with cancer wants to hear about all the people you know who've died from cancer. They're fighting for their lives. Trust me, they know every statistic, they know what their five-year survival probability is, and they understand on a very visceral level that, even if their treatments are successful, their cancer can come back and kill them.

They don't need a reminder.

What can you say instead? Maybe something like, "Wow, that's really scary. If you need someone to talk to about it, I'm here." Let the person with cancer—if they so choose—guide the conversation about their fears, hopes, and experiences. One of the best things you can do to support a person with cancer is to listen.

Then, similar to #2, there's "You're lucky. Some people have it way worse." I *think* it's meant to make the person with cancer think positively, but it's actually just toxic. *Of course* some people have it worse. Someone always has it better, and someone always has it worse. But it's not a contest. Trauma is trauma, and illness is illness, so don't diminish the real pain and suffering a person with cancer may be enduring by telling them to cheer up because it could be worse. Instead, if speaking to a person with cancer who has disclosed a good prognosis, say something like, "I'm so glad that you're going to be okay, but if you're not okay right now, I'm here for you. Cancer is cancer, and it must be hard." Invite them to share what they're going through—if they want to—and listen.

Remember Jon Stewart. When in doubt, don't be douchey.

You know those people who always have to make everything about them? That's what we're dealing with when it comes to #7. "Oh no— I've always been terrified that I would get cancer!" Yeah, I had a family member say that to me. *When I had cancer.* I called her out, and she got super offended at my insensitivity to her phobias. She legit has mental-health issues, but I do too, and I don't make it a fucking contest. If ever there were an occasion for saying "Bitch, please," this was it. Cancer is awful, and no one wants to get it. And it's totally okay to fear getting cancer. Feelings are feelings, and you cope with them and process them—but *not* with a person who actually has cancer. Again, talk to friends, family, or a therapist, but don't bring that baggage to a person who's already dealing with enough baggage, thanks to cancer. They have enough to carry.

And now we come to #8, the catchphrase of the toxic positivity vibe, "Stay positive!" On the surface, this seems like sage advice. A good mindset and positive outlook can help make many situations more bearable. But there's a flip side, a dark side, that's, well, toxic. According to Dr. Jaime Zuckerman, a psychologist who specializes in anxiety and self-esteem issues, "Toxic positivity is the assumption, either by one's self or others, that, despite a person's emotional pain or difficult situation, they should only have a positive mindset or—my pet peeve term—'positive vibes.'"[3] When people tell you to focus on the positives and be grateful that you're alive, or to change your outlook and choose happiness, it can come across as gaslighting. It can encourage the person who has cancer to suppress their real and valid negative emotions rather than processing them in a healthy way. It invalidates their experiences by pressuring the person to put on a brave face and pretend to be okay.

That's not helpful, and no good comes from suppressing normal emotions. Also, this kind of terrible advice can come from a place of selfishness on the part of the toxic-positivity cheerleader, who may not be comfortable with the grief, pain, depression, or anxiety experienced by the person with cancer. If you're not comfortable or are on overload—which happens, especially with caregivers—take a break. You need it! But do not assume the person with cancer has the obligation to put on a brave or happy face just to make you feel better.

It's not about you.

Dr. Elizabeth Yuko, bioethicist, provides some tips for dealing with toxic positivity on both the giving and receiving ends. Don't suppress or ignore your feelings, even if they're negative. Listen to and validate the experiences of others. Keep your unsolicited advice to yourself. Don't shame people or yourself for your emotions. Know that it's okay and normal to feel bad sometimes. Understand that you can experience many emotions all at once and that they're okay, even if they're conflicting. Be realistic about processing emotions and the experience, and don't give yourself a short deadline. And take a break from social media if that would be helpful.[4]

Sound advice on all fronts. Take it.

This next one, #9, also relates to toxic positivity. "You're so strong/brave. You've got this!" Whenever someone calls me brave or strong because I had cancer, I cringe. To me, bravery and strength come from actively fighting for things I believe in. The fight comes with risk, it requires courage, and, most importantly, it's something I *chose*. I didn't choose cancer. Nobody chooses cancer. As far as, "You've got this!" do I? One of the most terrible things about cancer is that it leaves the person with the disease feeling helpless. Someone operates on you, someone irradiates you, someone pumps chemotherapy into you, someone gives you daily meds, and it can leave you feeling like a passive bystander. I hate not being in charge or in control. Cancer steals your control. My health-care team is in charge; yes, they loop me in, and it's ultimately my decision which course to take, but I play no real active role in my treatments.

I'm not knocking the cancer warriors. Do whatever helps you get through and makes you feel empowered! But remember that it's okay to feel powerless, and it's okay to admit to yourself that you need help. As far as bravery, I usually tell people, "You'd be surprised what you can do when you have no choice." It's not deflection; I love praise as much as the next person. But to take credit for being courageous when I've spent hours curled in a ball and crying just feels . . . disingenuous. But

I'll take praise for putting long hours in the lab that have left me curled in a ball and crying; that was my choice and my fight.

Instead of being a pathologically enthusiastic cheerleader, maybe instead say, "This must be scary to go through. That's okay. Know you're not alone and that it's okay to ask for help or talk about the scary stuff." Believe me, this is super comforting. I cherish the friends and family who've approached these difficult conversations by validating how I feel and inviting me to talk about it.

Finally, #10, "God never gives you more than you can handle." First off, not everyone believes in your god or *a* god, so don't assume. Second, this sentiment smacks of "these things happen for a reason," like some higher power is testing you or punishing you. Very Old Testament, and not very helpful for someone with cancer. Again, the person with cancer is likely railing at the universe and asking, "Why me?" They don't need you telling them that it was the will of your god that they be tested.

My advice is going to piss some people off, but so be it.

Faith can be a wonderful thing, and many people facing cancer find comfort, solace, and hope in their faith and in their communities of faith. These communities can offer support in the form of prayers and should also offer actionable help in the form of caring for the person with cancer and their family and by providing assistance with their needs like food, childcare, or financial assistance. That can be one of the most beautiful aspects of faith—acts of service and love. Emphasis on *acts*. Just saying "I'll pray for you" to someone with cancer is an empty platitude, even if it's sincere.

Pray all you want, but I'd really appreciate a casserole and a shoulder to cry on.

If the person with cancer says they believe that "God's got this," then it's their prerogative. I've heard this sentiment sincerely expressed by many survivor sisters, and I'm so glad that it brings them comfort and strength. But no one else should make that assumption or say that to them. It's douchey. Don't be douchey.

And here's a bonus! #11, "What can I do?" Okay, on the surface, it's really sweet when you ask what the person needs or what you can do for them. It's not always the wrong thing to say. But here's the thing—the person with cancer is already overwhelmed with so much, so asking them to come up with things for you to do can feel like just one more thing that they have to do. If you're like me, it's really hard to accept help. My automatic default is, "Thanks, but I'm good," even when I'm not good. It's knee-jerk, it's part of my upbringing, and it's a handy way to get out of feeling put on the spot. Instead, ask the *caregiver* or *family* of the person with cancer what you can do. Or you can drop food off for the person's family. Having meals ready to eat is such a relief—believe me. The last thing I or anyone in my house wanted to do after surgeries and treatments was cook or think about picking up dinner. Offer the caregiver your services for running errands and for being a point of contact for other concerned friends and family so the caregiver and person with cancer isn't constantly answering phone calls, texts, or emails. Offer the caregiver your services for childcare, dropping kids off at school or picking them up, or driving the person with cancer to and from appointments.

Even something as simple as a shared meme or GIF on social media is a nice, no-pressure way to let the person with cancer know you're thinking of them.

Next up, I'll cover moving forward in life post–breast cancer—or in life *with* breast cancer—with humor and hope. This chapter includes practical advice, perspective, and some of the really incredible advances that are being made in breast cancer prevention and treatment. It's an exciting time in the field, and there are some game changers with real promise just around the corner. And that's not toxic positivity, either. It's real, and it's wonderful.

~

CHAPTER SIXTEEN

Life Goes On

Moving Forward with Humor and Hope

Survivorship and life postcancer is something that's still very new for me. While my status is no evidence of disease (NED), I'm not actually finished with breast reconstruction. As of this writing, I'm projected to need two more revision surgeries to match my left reconstructed breast to my right in terms of size and overall appearance. As far as treatments go, I'll be taking estrogen blockers for the next seven years, for a total of ten years, and I'll likely be in medically induced menopause through Lupron injections for another three years, for a total of five years. It's like a freakin' prison term.

This is my normal, and I think about my breast cancer every single day.

I look forward to the day when I don't think about it as much—assuming that day comes. It may not. But it's not going to hold me hostage or take over my life. I won't let it. I'll fight breast cancer on the fronts I did before—in the laboratory—as well as in the public arena as an advocate for science, health equity, and health equality. I'll keep fighting in the political sphere as an advocate for research funding and patient care. I'll fight in the blogosphere and bookiverse to spread information and debunk scams, misinformation, and all things pseudo-science. That's what I think survivorship and life after breast cancer will look like for me.

What will it look like for you if you're a patient or survivor? That's up to you. There are no right or wrong paths. You don't have to have some grand mission or newfound purpose. It's good to find a way to process the emotions that come along with the experience. For me, writing has proven to be very helpful. Making art, connecting with friends and family in a deeper way, and finding joy and gratitude in quiet moments or in milestones are all meaningful paths forward. Hopefully you'll come out on the other side with the ability to recognize what's important to you versus what's just background noise. I've found it very liberating to let go of worries about my career progress and about whether or not I'm good enough as a human being, as a mother, as a friend, as a daughter, as a wife. *I am*. You're good enough too. Give yourself permission to quit sweating the small stuff and focus on what matters most to you. Embrace that. Enjoy that. Life is too short to waste on the noise, and it's too beautiful to neglect the good stuff.

I also recommend laughter. Find the funny whenever and wherever you can, and laugh until your sides hurt and tears roll down your face. Belly laughs are the best (unless you have stitches; hold off until those are out).

Since no one can really be objective about themselves, I asked my family how they think cancer has changed me for good or ill. According to my husband, the way I presented myself to the world during cancer was positive and even-keeled. He said many people told him they were amazed at how well I was handling it all, though he knew better than anyone else about my struggles, doubts, anger, frustration, and darkness. Basically, I'm good at masking. That's not necessarily a good thing. I don't want to be the poster girl for toxic positivity. What these people didn't see was how I fell apart in private. If they pick up a copy of this book and read chapter 8, they'll realize that I'm not superhuman. I'm neurotic and nerdy—but in an entertaining way! That's good. Patrick also told me that now I'm more decisive after cancer; I know what I want and what I don't want, and I'm not afraid to say no. That's fair—and a good thing. He also noted that I'm freer. I don't stress about the small stuff in life. I've got my priorities in line. That's a good thing.

My daughter is glad that I kept my sense of humor. I'm glad too.

My son is glad I'm alive. Me too, buddy. Me, too.

There will be good days and dark nights of the soul that you will navigate—good days where you hardly think about cancer at all and bad days where you sit in a waiting room, heart racing or sinking, hoping that your follow-up scan is clear and terrified that it isn't. I think about that a lot, especially since something has come up on every mammogram I've ever had. What if it comes back? It may. I was relatively young when I got my diagnosis, so any breast cancer cells sitting dormant in my body will have more time to wake up and wreak havoc. They'll have more time to acquire more mutations and alterations that can make them stronger and more deadly. I had one positive lymph node, so my risk of distant recurrence after twenty years is 20 percent. Risk of death due to distant recurrence after twenty years is 13 percent.[1] It's a sobering thought. Is there anything I can do about it? Other than take my meds and try to live a healthy lifestyle, it's really out of my hands. It's chaos.

I'll be kind.

I'll also take comfort in the fact that we're getting new weapons in the arsenal for fighting breast cancer. Antitumor immunity is the hottest thing to hit the field of cancer research since the 2001 approval of Gleevec (a game-changer drug used to treat chronic myelogenous leukemia that targets the oncoprotein product of the Philadelphia chromosome that drives the disease) and the 2006 approval of Gardasil (first vaccine targeting the human papilloma virus strains that cause most cervical cancers). Recently *Frontiers in Immunology* published the history of antitumor immunity efforts leading to the development of immune-checkpoint inhibitors available in the clinic today, the use of engineered T-cells taken from patients and altered to fight their cancer, and oncolytic viruses.[2] I'll go over the basics, including how antitumor immunity works and the challenges we still face in getting tumors to respond.

Before we get into how antitumor immunity works, we need to understand how the immune system works to fight infection. It's a complex beast, but here are some basics. Your immune system functions to mount a rapid and robust defense when your body encounters a pathogen (e.g., a virus or bacteria that causes disease) in your daily life. The arm of the immune system that does this is called the *adaptive immune system* (figure 16.1). The other arm is the *innate immune system*, which includes natural barriers like skin, the tiny hairs and mucous in your nose, and stomach acid. The adaptive immune system is what antitumor immunity treatments harness. It is also altered by tumors to suppress tumor immune responses and exploited to work for the tumor. (More on that in a bit.)

The adaptive immune system works like this: Specialized cells iden- tify a potential threat (e.g., an infection), and they carry information about that threat in the form of bits of protein called *antigens* to other immune cells. If the threat is credible, those immune cells get activated

Adaptive immune system

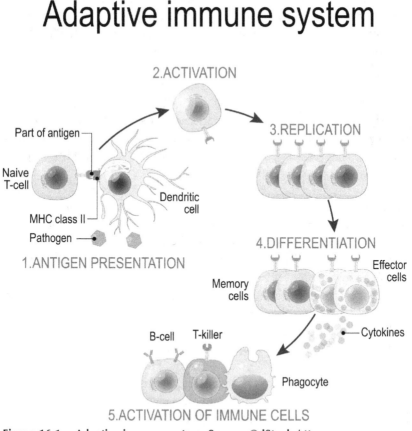

Figure 16.1.   Adaptive immune system. *Source:* © iStock / ttsz.

and fight the threat. First the specialized cells that identify a potential threat patrol your body, looking for something suspicious. Cells like macrophages and dendritic cells, which roam around various organs and tissues, find *pathogens* (a bacteria, virus, or other microbe that causes disease) or unhealthy cells infected by pathogens, and eat them (the fancy term is *phagocytosis*). Infected or damaged cells send out protein signals called *cytokines* as a distress call to attract these patrolling macrophages and dendritic cells. While "digesting" the bacteria or infected cell, macrophages and dendritic cells salvage proteins or pieces of proteins—*antigens*—that identify the bacteria or virus as "other," and they present these to immune cells, usually in lymph nodes, which in turn mount an immune response. Macrophages and dendritic cells are known as professional *antigen presenting cells* (APCs).

When activated by APCs, immune cells called *B-cells* produce *antibodies* against the antigen, which can do a lot of things to fight an infection. Some antibodies neutralize the pathogen by binding it and stopping it from entering a cell. Other antibodies tag infected cells as a signal for other immune cells to come and kill them. Others coat pathogens or infected cells in a process called *opsonization* (meaning "the process of making tasty"), which signals other cells like macrophages to come and eat the coated pathogens or cells. Specialized B-cells called *memory B-cells* store the information about the antigen so your immune system can recognize the pathogen when it hits you again and mount a faster immune response.

Other immune cells called *T-cells*, which are particularly relevant to antitumor immunity, become activated by APCs and mount a different kind of immune response. *Cytotoxic T-cells* seek out and kill infected or damaged cells, and *helper T-cells* help activate B-cells so they make antibodies, activate cytotoxic T-cells, and activate macrophages to go eat nasty invaders and infected cells. *Memory T-cells* also store information about past infections to mount a rapid, strong response the next time your body sees them.

That's a simplified but hopefully digestible explanation of immunity and the major players (there are other immune cells, but APCs, B-cells, and T-cells are the biggies).

Memory is key to protection, and memory is built by exposure to pathogens.

Put a pin in that concept for when we get to anticancer vaccines, and also remember what T-cells do for when we get to engineered CAR T-cells and oncolytic viruses.

Working out how to harness your body's own immune system to fight cancer isn't a new idea. It's been under investigation since the nineteenth century. In fact, in chapter 5 we covered the way trastuzumab (trade name Herceptin), a humanized anti-HER2 antibody, targets HER2-expressing breast cancer cells for death. Herceptin and other monoclonal antibodies mimic the natural activity of antibody-producing B-cells to deliver therapies and tag cancer antigen–expressing cells for immune-mediated destruction. But it was the discovery of checkpoint inhibitors—proteins that put T-cells in a state of exhaustion and inactivity in pathways that are exploited by many cancers—that led to the first molecularly targeted therapies designed to boost antitumor immunity. Doctors James Allison and Tasuku Honjo pioneered this Nobel Prize–winning work.[3]

What are immune-checkpoint inhibitors, and how do they work? T-cells, particularly cytotoxic T-cells that actively kill their targets, bind to antigens on tumor cells through their T-cell receptors. But tumor cells, being the adaptable beasts that they are, can produce proteins like PD-L1 (programmed death ligand 1), which bind to PD-1 (programmed cell death protein 1), proteins on T-cells. This interaction tells the T-cell to stand down by tricking it into thinking that the tumor cell is "self" and should be protected. Signaling networks like this normally promote self-tolerance so that your immune system doesn't attack your own healthy cells (figure 16.2). In tumors, it works by telling tumor-infiltrating T-cells, if present, to go into a state of inactivity. Drugs that target PD-L1—like atezolizumab (trade name Tecentriq), durvalumab (trade name Imfinzi), and avelumab (trade name Bavencio)—and drugs that target PD-1—like nivolumab (trade name Opdivo) and pembrolizumab (trade name Keytruda)—are FDA-approved monoclonal-antibody therapies that block interactions between PD-1/PD-L1 to unleash an antitumor immune response.[4]

Other immune-checkpoint molecules exploited by cancers include cytotoxic T lymphocyte antigen 4 (CTLA-4), the target of the first FDA-approved immune-checkpoint inhibitor ipilimumab (trade name Yervoy). Approved in 2011 for advanced melanoma, this drug had

T-cell

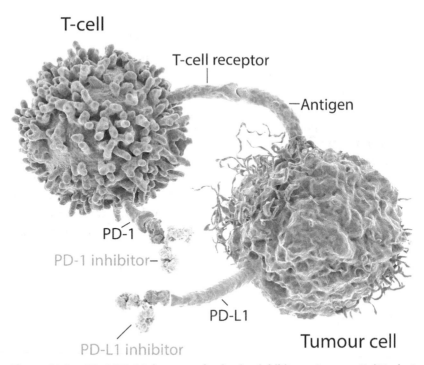

Figure 16.2.   PD-1/PD-L1 immune-checkpoint inhibitors. *Source:* © iStock / Dr_Microbe.

remarkable results. In fact, over 20 percent of the patients enrolled in the initial ipilimumab clinical trials (before the 2011 approval) are still alive and show no evidence of disease (NED).

There's some incredible potential in targeting checkpoint inhibitors.

CTLA-4 is part of a cellular-signaling pathway that normally fine-tunes immune responses. CTLA-4 and a similar receptor, CD28, are expressed on two different T-cell types: (1) CD4+ helper T-cells, which help activate other immune cells to mediate adaptive immune responses, and (2) CD8+ cytotoxic T-cells, those cells that kill infected cells, damaged cells, and, if properly activated, tumor cells. Antigen-presenting cells make a protein called B7, which can bind to either CD28 or CTLA-4 on T-cells, and the effects on T-cell function are very different depending on what B7 binds. If it binds to CD28, B7 activates T-cell responses as a part of a complex of proteins that includes the T-cell receptor. Binding of B7 to CTLA-4 shuts down T-cell functions. CTLA-4 probably serves as protection from self-antigen recognition by inducing immune suppression, since laboratory mouse models engineered to *not* express CTLA-4 die from autoimmunity. This is the aspect of CTLA-4 function that gets highjacked by tumor cells. Drugs like ipilimumab block the suppressive activity of CTLA-4, which can allow T-cells to attack tumor cells.[5]

Here's the kicker: The tumor actually has to have infiltrating T-cells for this to work, and not all tumors do. Tumors with T-cells that can be activated to fight the tumor are called "hot," whereas tumors without T-cells are "cold." One of the most aggressively researched topics in tumor immunology right now is how to make a cold tumor hot and thus responsive to antitumor immune therapies.

This is especially important for breast cancer, since most subtypes produce cold tumors. Right now, immune-checkpoint therapies are only approved for advanced triple-negative breast cancers that make the PD-L1 protein. Not all triple-negative breast cancers make PD-L1. Ongoing research is looking to expand the use of immune therapy in inflammatory breast cancer and the HER2+ subtype.[6] Hopefully, with more research, we'll figure out how to make more tumors responsive to immune therapy by making them hot (full of T-cells) and by discovering other immune checkpoints that can be targeted.

New therapies designed to induce or boost antitumor immunity also need to overcome the ability of tumor cells to trick the body into suppressing immunity. Tumor cells are adaptive, and they're also sneaky little bastards, altering their metabolism (e.g., how they process nutrients) and changing their cell-surface proteins to suppress immune responses against them. They can even change the nature of immune-cell components, like making macrophages work for them instead of alerting the immune system to the threat of cancer cells, and can recruit cells called myeloid-derived suppressor cells (MDSCs), which thwart immune responses. We also need to reduce the risk that cancer patients treated with immune-checkpoint inhibitors or other immune therapies don't develop autoimmune disorders as a side effect. Remember, cancer cells come from normal cells in our bodies, so there's a risk that the immune system will inadvertently respond to a self-antigen on tumors that will lead to attacks on normal cells that also express it.

Working around these clever tricks that tumors use to block antitumor immunity is a challenge, but understanding how the system works will create new opportunities for drug and therapy development.

Another way to harness the power of the body's immune system to fight cancer is the use of engineered T-cells. Chimeric antigen receptor (CAR) T-cell therapy is currently used to treat blood cancers, and it works like this: T-cells are isolated from the patient's blood, purified to get rid of non-T-cells, and grown in the laboratory. Autologous-antigen-presenting cells (APCs from the patient) are also purified and cultured with the T-cells, and cytokines that polarize and activate the T-cells that are added to the mix.[7] The cells are maintained in a culture dish and genetically engineered to make T-cell receptors that recognize antigens on cancer cells. The genetic material for modified T-cell receptors is delivered by viruses that are used as vectors (e.g., viruses that infect T-cells and introduce genetic material designed in a lab but that doesn't cause a disease) or by other laboratory methods.[8] The modified cells are then infused back into the patient, where they will hopefully mount a response against tumor cells expressing the antigen that the T-cell receptor was designed to target.

Barriers to use right now include expense and the fact that engineered T-cells haven't worked as well in solid tumors like breast cancers. Solid tumor cells tend to lose antigen expression, so the engineered T-cells can no longer recognize them, or else the solid tumor cells tend to lack unique antigens that distinguish them from normal healthy cells. Also the immune-suppressive environment created by many solid tumors makes it difficult for CAR-T cells to work.[9] New strategies—like using gene-editing technology to construct multitarget CAR-T cells that recognize multiple antigens, and enhancing CAR-T cell growth and the longevity of these cells by causing the cells to make costimulatory proteins and cytokines that boost T-cell growth and function—are being tested to broaden the use of these cells to more cancer types. Also, gene editing is being used to delete immune-checkpoint-inhibitor proteins in these T-cells to prevent suppression by tumor cells.[10]

Another very recent and exciting development is the use of anti-cancer vaccines, which have just entered clinical trials for some breast cancer subtypes. Remember how your adaptive immune system works? Patrolling antigen-presenting cells pick up bits and pieces of proteins from infected or damaged cells, take them to other immune cells, and then mount a defense. This is what happens when you get infected with pathogens like viruses that can make you very sick in the process. After your body is exposed to a pathogen and mounts an immune response, it "remembers" the pathogen by maintaining memory B-cells and T-cells that recognize the antigen and can fight the pathogen more effectively if you're exposed to it again.

But what if there were a way to expose your body to pathogens *without* making you sick? That's where vaccines come in!

Vaccines work by tapping into this process to activate the adaptive immune response using an *artificial antigen* supplied by the vaccine, getting your immune response geared up and, importantly, building up archival memory B- and T-cells that will recognize the real infection when your body encounters it so it can rapidly fight it. The vaccine basically creates a mock infection without the getting-sick part. Types of vaccines include live-attenuated vaccines, inactivated vaccines, toxoid vaccines, and subunit, recombinant, polysaccharide, and conjugate vaccines.[11]

- *Live-attenuated* means using a weakened form of the virus to initiate an immune response; examples include the measles, mumps, and rubella (MMR) vaccine and the chickenpox vaccine.
- *Inactivated* means using a dead version of the virus that cannot infect cells but contains antigens that can be used to activate adaptive immunity; examples include flu, hepatitis A, and rabies vaccines.
- *Toxoid* vaccines use toxins produced by the pathogen to mount an immune response against the toxic protein; examples include tetanus and diphtheria vaccines.
- *Subunit, recombinant, polysaccharide,* and *conjugate* vaccines use pieces of the virus that act as antigens, like proteins and sugars; examples include HPV, hepatitis B, and shingles vaccines.
- Newer vaccines, like those developed by Pfizer and Moderna against SARS-CoV-2, the virus that causes COVID-19, work by delivering mRNA that encodes the spike-protein antigen from

the virus. Your own cells then translate the mRNA into protein, and your immune system is alerted and mounts an adaptive response against it without you getting sick.[12]

As I mentioned earlier, an anticancer vaccine was developed to combat the human papilloma virus that ended up reducing the incidence of cervical cancer by 90 percent in vaccinated women, which shows the power of vaccines in cancer prevention.[13] The FDA approved a vaccine targeting triple-negative breast cancer for clinical trials in 2020.[14] The vaccine target is a protein called alpha-lactalbumin, which is expressed by many breast cancer cells of the triple-negative subtype. The first trial will be a Phase I trial, designed to test the safety of the vaccine. Since alpha-lactalbumin is a milk protein, the vaccine could disrupt milk production and will not be tested on women who intend to breast feed. If the vaccine is successful, it will be interesting to see how the vaccine would be used. It's preventative, so should all women receive it (maybe not given the effects on breastfeeding), or should it only be offered to high-risk patients? The same questions will likely apply for vaccines in the clinical pipeline, including those against the HER2 oncoprotein for HER2+ breast cancer and a vaccine against mammaglobin-A, which is expressed in a broader subset of breast cancers and showed promising results in an early Phase I trial.[15] Another ongoing Phase I trial is testing the safety of a modified measles-virus vaccine carrier designed to express neutrophil-activating protein, which stimulates the patient's immune system and enhances anticancer immune responses. In preclinical laboratory studies (laboratory mouse models), the vaccine boosted immune responses to breast cancers regardless of their HER2 and hormone-receptor status.[16]

These studies are so promising and give me so much hope. Between all the other studies testing small-molecule inhibitors, new technologies harnessing nanoparticles and carriers as well as peptides designed to deliver siRNA therapy or other drugs, and other discoveries being made in laboratories all over the world that we haven't even heard of yet (but we will), it's an amazing time to be a cancer researcher and a hopeful time for patients and survivors. Having been on both sides, it's hope that drives me, inspires me, and keeps me going in the laboratory, in science outreach and patient advocacy, and in life.

In spite of the uncertainty that's always there, my adventure continues, and for that I'm profoundly grateful.

Speaking of adventures . . . I'm very much a work in progress in terms of breast reconstruction. Over the course of three years, my boobs have migrated at least three inches up my chest and have changed size and shape along the way. Want to see? I've only ever seen the end product when I've surfed plastic-surgery galleries, so I thought it might be useful for folks to see the intermediate stages for some of these surgical interventions.

(Dad, please feel free to skip this part, but know that this is for educational and medical purposes.)

Here's the before picture (figure 16.3), my original breasts at forty-five years old—size 38D and a bit saggy, but I loved them. And I miss them. They were mine. This is the last time I saw them as they were, on May 11, 2018, just before my lumpectomy and oncoplastic surgery.

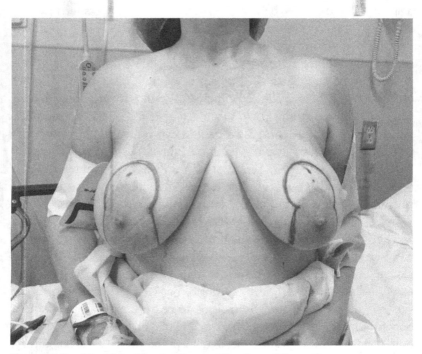

Figure 16.3. My original boobs. *Source:* Courtesy of the author.

Fast forward to 2019, one year after surgery and radiation treatments, and here are my new boobs (figure 16.4). With the reduction and lift part of the oncoplastic reconstruction, I became a 38C. The shape is gorgeous, and aside from keloid scarring around and below my right nipple and radiation damage on the left (which isn't as visible as much as it is tactile), they're damned near perfect.

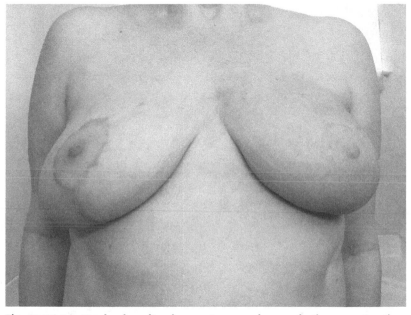

Figure 16.4. My boobs after lumpectomy and oncoplastic reconstruction. *Source:* Courtesy of the author.

About a year after that, I said goodbye to the left breast, thanks to residual disease, and prior to reconstruction I had a small expander. Here's how I looked after a few fills in the expander (figure 16.5). The left side with the expander is much higher than the right breast. (Honestly, I look a little bit like a Picasso.) Thankfully, it was only temporary!

In November of 2020, I had my DUG flap reconstruction. It looked better for sure (figure 16.6). The left side has the graft but not as much volume. The right got a lift and a bit of a reduction as part of the

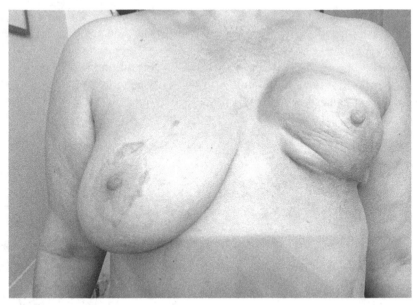

Figure 16.5.   My boobs after mastectomy. *Source:* Courtesy of the author.

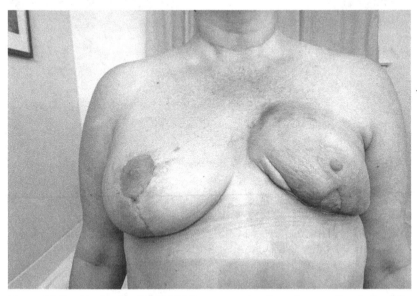

Figure 16.6.   My boobs after DUG flap reconstruction. *Source:* Courtesy of the author.

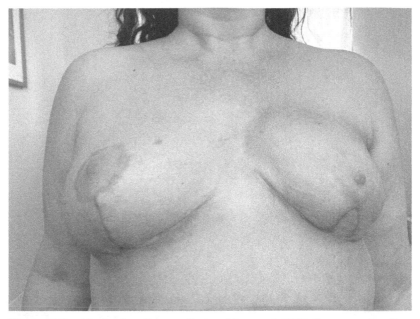

Figure 16.7. My boobs after my first revision post–DUG flap reconstruction. *Source:* Courtesy of the author.

matching process. As you can see, it's a process. The revisions, which consist of a series of fat grafts, will add volume and hopefully better match them.

Here's where I'm at now, in March of 2021, after my first revision (figure 16.7). It gets better. I'm hopeful. And grateful. And happy.

~

Appendix

Aesthetic flat closure, Not Putting On a Shirt, https://notputting
onashirt.org/
American Association for Cancer Research, https://www.aacr
.org/
American Association of Sexuality Educators, Counselors and
Therapists, https://www.aasect.org/
American Cancer Society, https://www.cancer.org/
Animal research
  "How Mouse Models Pave the Way to Precision Cancer Med-
  icine," American Association for Cancer Research press
  office, AACR.org blog, September 21, 2019, https://www
  .aacr.org/blog/2017/09/21/how-mouse-models-pave-the-way
  -to-precision-cancer-medicine/.
  "Medical Benefits," Speaking of Research (website), accessed
  June 18, 2021, https://speakingofresearch.com/facts/medical
  -benefits/.
  Office of Laboratory Animal Welfare (OLAW), https://olaw
  .nih.gov/home.htm
  Institutional Animal Care and Use Committees (IACUC),
  https://www.aalas.org/iacuc

American Association for Laboratory Animal Science (AALAS), https://www.aalas.org/
Antitumor immunity
"The Intriguing History of Cancer Immunotherapy," Paula Do-bosz and Tomasz Dzieciątkowski in *Frontiers in Immunology* 10 (December 17, 2019): 2965, https://www.frontiersin.org/articles/10.3389/fimmu.2019.02965/full.
"Immunotherapy for Breast Cancer," American Cancer Society medical and editorial content team, Treating Breast Cancer, American Cancer Society, Cancer.org, last revised December 3, 2020, https://www.cancer.org/cancer/breast-cancer/treatment/immunotherapy.html.
Asian American Cancer Support Network, http://aacsn.org/
Black breast cancer–patient support
Sisters Network, Inc., http://www.sistersnetworkinc.org/
The African American Healthcare Alliance, https://www.aahafortwayne.org/
Sisters by Choice, https://www.sistersbychoice.org/
Black Women's Health Imperative, https://bwhi.org/
2for2 Boobs, https://2for2boobs.org/
Black excellence in cancer research and medicine: BlackinCancer, https://www.blackincancer.com/
BRCA genes: "BRCA: The Breast Cancer Gene, " National Breast Cancer Foundation, Inc., last reviewed April 15, 2020, https://www.nationalbreastcancer.org/what-is-brca.
Breast biology and breast cancer: *What You Need to Know about Breast Cancer*, National Cancer Institute booklet, NIH publication no. 12-1556, revised August 2012, https://pubs.cancer.gov/pdf/Insides-wyntk-breast.pdf.
Breast cancer—men: "Breast Cancer in Men," Centers for Disease Control and Prevention, CDC.gov, last reviewed August 11, 2020, https://www.cdc.gov/cancer/breast/men/index.htm.
Breast cancer—research funding
National Cancer Institute (NCI), https://www.cancer.gov/
National Institutes of Health (NIH), https://www.nih.gov/
Congressionally Directed Medical Research Programs (CDMRP) under the Department of Defense (DOD), https://cdmrp.army.mil/

Breast cancer risk factors

"What Are the Risk Factors for Breast Cancer?" Centers for Disease Control and Prevention, CDC.gov, last reviewed September 14, 2020, https://www.cdc.gov/cancer/breast/basic _info/risk_factors.htm.

"Hormones," National Institutes of Health, National Cancer Institute, Cancer.gov, April 29, 2015, https://www.cancer.gov/ about-cancer/causes-prevention/risk/hormones.

"Using HRT (Hormone Replacement Therapy)," Breastcancer. org, last modified April 21, 2021, https://www.breastcancer. org/risk/factors/hrt.

Breast Cancer Facts and Figures, 2019–2020, American Cancer Society (Atlanta: American Cancer Society, Inc., 2019), https:// www.cancer.org/content/dam/cancer-org/research/cancer -facts-and-statistics/breast-cancer-facts-and-figures/breast-can- cer-facts-and-figures-2019-2020.pdf.

Breast cancer subtypes

"Types," National Breast Cancer Foundation, Inc., last reviewed April 15, 2020, https://www.nationalbreastcancer.org/types-of- breast-cancer/.

"Cancer Stat Facts: Female Breast Cancer Subtypes," National Cancer Institute, Surveillance, Epidemiology, and End Results Program, accessed June 25, 2021, https://seer.cancer.gov/stat facts/html/breast-subtypes.html.

"A Disease with Many Faces," David R. Hout, Diagnostics, *The Pathologist*, May 3, 2019, https://thepathologist.com/ diagnostics/a-disease-with-many-faces.

"Breast Self-Exam," Breastcancer.org, last modified October 24, 2019, https://www.breastcancer.org/symptoms/testing/types/self_ exam.

Cancer biology

"What Is Cancer?" CancerQuest, Emory University, Winship Cancer Institute, accessed June 25, 2021, http://www.cancer quest.org/patients/what-cancer.

"Why We Haven't Cured Cancer," *SciShow*, video, uploaded May 14, 2015, https://www.youtube.com/watch?v=7tzaWOdvGMw.

"Cancer as an Evolutionary Process: Clonal Evolution," Yale-Course, video, uploaded May 14, 2014, https://www.youtube.com/watch?v=wH9jmQglOLw.

"Metastasis: How Cancer Spreads," National Cancer Institute, National Institutes of Health, US Department of Health and Human Services, December 2016, https://www.youtube.com/watch?v=fQwar_-QdiQ.

"Hereditary Breast Cancer and BRCA Genes," Centers for Disease Control and Prevention, CDC.gov, last reviewed April 5, 2019, https://www.cdc.gov/cancer/breast/young_women/bringyourbrave/hereditary_breast_cancer/.

Cannabis cancer-therapy side effects

"7 Uses and Benefits of CBD Oil (Plus Side Effects)," Jillian Kubala for *Healthline*, February 26, 2018. https://www.healthline.com/nutrition/cbd-oil-benefits.

"Cannabis and Cannabinoids (PDQ®)–Health Professional Version," National Institutes of Health, National Cancer Institute, Cancer.gov, updated June 3, 2021, https://www.cancer.gov/about-cancer/treatment/cam/hp/cannabis-pdq.

"Clinical Trials Using Marijuana," National Cancer Institute, National Institutes of Health, Cancer.gov, accessed June 25, 2021, https://www.cancer.gov/about-cancer/treatment/clinical-trials/intervention/marijuana.

"The Central Dogma: From Genomic Information to Protein Synthesis," RIKEN Omics Science Center, video, made as part of the Beyond Genetics exhibit at the National Science Museum of Japan, 2007, https://www.youtube.com/watch?v=-ygpqVr7_xs.

Chemotherapy

Chemotherapy and You: Support for People with Cancer, National Cancer Institute, NIH publication no. 18-7157 ([Washington, DC]: US Department of Health and Human Services and the National Cancer Institute Office of Communications and Public Liaison, 2018), https://www.cancer.gov/publications/patient-education/chemotherapy-and-you.pdf.

"How Is Chemotherapy Given?" Breastcancer.org, last modified March 25, 2020, https://www.breastcancer.org/treatment/chemotherapy/process/how.

"Chemotherapy for Breast Cancer," Mayo Clinic staff, May-Clinic.org, February 24, 2021, https://www.mayoclinic.org/tests-procedures/chemotherapy-for-breast-cancer/about/pac-20384931.

"Chemo Brain," American Cancer Society medical and editorial team, Cancer.org, last revised February 1, 2020, https://www.cancer.org/treatment/treatments-and-side-effects/physical-side-effects/changes-in-mood-or-thinking/chemo-brain.html.

Chronic diseases

"About Chronic Diseases," Centers for Disease Control and Prevention, CDC.gov, last reviewed April 28, 2021, https://www.cdc.gov/chronicdisease/about/index.htm.

"Chronic Illness," Health Library, Cleveland Clinic, May 10, 2021, https://my.clevelandclinic.org/health/articles/4062-chronic-illness.

Cognitive behavioral therapy

"What Is Cognitive Behavioral Therapy?" American Psychological Association, APA.org, July 2017, https://www.apa.org/ptsd-guideline/patients-and-families/cognitive-behavioral.

"What Are Cognitive Distortions and How Can You Change These Thinking Patterns? 'Should' Statements," Rebecca Joy Stanborough for *Healthline*, December 18, 2019, https://www.healthline.com/health/cognitive-distortions#should-statements.

Complementary alternative medicine

"How Does Complementary Medicine Work?" Breastcancer.org, last modified May 5, 2020, https://www.breastcancer.org/treatment/comp_med/what_is_it/how_it_works.

"The Truth about Alternative Medical Treatments," American Cancer Society medical and editorial content team, Cancer.org, January 30, 2019, https://www.cancer.org/latest-news/the-truth-about-alternative-medical-treatments.html.

Connecting with survivors

Reach to Recovery, https://reach.cancer.org/

"Support Groups," Breastcancer.org, last modified May 5, 2020, https://www.breastcancer.org/treatment/comp_med/types/group.

"Breast Cancer Support Group," National Breast Cancer Foundation, Inc., accessed June 25, 2021, https://www.national breastcancer.org/nbcf-programs/breast-cancer-support-group.

Cancer Support Community, https://www.cancersupportcom munity.org/

Disabled breast cancer–patient support

The American Association of People with Disabilities, https:// www.aapd.com/

American Association on Intellectual and Developmental Disabilities, https://www.aaidd.org/

Disparities in cancer

"Cancer Disparities," National Institutes of Health, National Cancer Institute, Cancer.gov, updated November 17, 2020, https:// www.cancer.gov/about-cancer/understanding/disparities.

"Reducing Disparities in Health Care," Patient Support and Advocacy, American Medical Association, accessed June 17, 2021, https://www.ama-assn.org/delivering-care/patient -support-advocacy/reducing-disparities-health-care.

"Cultural Competence Training for Health Care Professionals," County Health Rankings (website), University of Wisconsin Population Health Institute, last updated January 17, 2020, https://www.countyhealthrankings.org/take-action -to-improve-health/what-works-for-health/strategies/cultural -competence-training-for-health-care-professionals.

"Basic and Translational Disparities Research Funding," National Cancer Institute, National Institutes of Health, Cancer. gov, updated January 13, 2021, https://www.cancer.gov/about -nci/organization/crchd/disparities-research/basic-research.

"Fibroadenoma," American Society of Breast Surgeons, Breast360 .org, accessed June 17, 2021, https://breast360.org/topic/2015/ 10/24/fibroadenoma/.

Financial-assistance resources

"Susan G. Komen Treatment Assistance Program," Susan G. Komen (organization), Komen.org, August 2020, https://www .komen.org/wp-content/uploads/2020-Komen-TAP-Helpline -Flyer-Eng-Aug-2.pdf.

"I've Just Been Diagnosed with Breast Cancer. Even with Insurance, I Have Many Out-of-Pocket Expenses. What Organizations

Can Help Me?'" answered by Jane Levy, Ask CancerCare Q&A, CancerCare.org, accessed June 25, 2021, https://www .cancercare.org/questions/136.

"Finding Financial Assistance," Metastatic Breast Cancer Network, MBCN.org, accessed June 25, 2021, http://mbcn.org/ finding-financial-assistance/.

"Additional Resources," Get Support, Living Beyond Breast Cancer (website), accessed June 25, 2021, https://www.lbbc .org/get-support/additional-resources

"Breast Cancer Assistance Program," American Breast Cancer Foundation, accessed June 25, 2021, https://www.abcf.org/pro grams/breast-cancer-assistance-program.

"FoundationOne®CDx," Foundation Medicine, accessed June 25, 2021, https://www.foundationmedicine.com/test/foundation one-cdx.

Gilda's Club, https://www.cancersupportcommunity.org

HER2-positive breast cancer

"Breast Cancer HER2 Status," American Cancer Society medical and editorial content team, Cancer.org, last revised September 20, 2019, https://www.cancer.org/cancer/breast -cancer/understanding-a-breast-cancer-diagnosis/breast-cancer -her2-status.html.

"HER2 Status," Breastcancer.org, last modified September 21, 2020, https://www.breastcancer.org/symptoms/diagnosis/her2.

"HER2+ Breast Cancer Survival Rates," Breast Cancer Guide, WebMD, last reviewed May 17, 2020, https://www.webmd .com/breast-cancer/guide/her2-positive-breast-cancer-survival -rates.

HER2-targeted therapies: "Herceptin Dosing and Administration," Herceptin.com, accessed March 15, 2021, https://www .herceptin.com/hcp/dosing-admin.html.

Hormone receptor–positive breast cancer

"Hormone Receptor Status," Breastcancer.org, last modified September 21, 2020, https://www.breastcancer.org/symptoms/ diagnosis/hormone_status.

"Breast Cancer HER2 Status," American Cancer Society medical and editorial content team, Cancer.org, last revised

September 20, 2019, https://www.cancer.org/cancer/breast
-cancer/understanding-a-breast-cancer-diagnosis/breast-cancer
-her2-status.html.

Hormone therapies

"How to Read Hormone Receptor Test Results," Breastcancer
.org, last modified September 21, 2020, https://www.breastcan
cer.org/symptoms/diagnosis/hormone_status/read_results.

"Lupron Depot® 7.5 Mg (Leuprolide Acetate for Depot Suspension)," US Food and Drug Administration, drug information
sheet, FDA.gov, October 7, 2011, https://www.accessdata
.fda.gov/drugsatfda_docs/label/2012/019732s038lbl.pdf.

"Evaluation of Lasofoxifene versus Fulvestrant in Advanced or
Metastatic ER+/HER2– Breast Cancer with an ESR1 Mutation," US National Library of Medicine, ClinicalTrials.gov,
National Institutes of Health, accessed June 18, 2021, https://
clinicaltrials.gov/ct2/show/NCT03781063.

"Hormone Therapy for Breast Cancer," American Cancer Society medical and editorial content team, Cancer.org, last
revised September 18, 2019, https://www.cancer.org/cancer/
breast-cancer/treatment/hormone-therapy-for-breast-cancer
.html.

Intraductal papilloma

"Intraductal Papilloma," Breast Cancer Now (website), last
reviewed December 2018, https://breastcancernow.org/infor
mation-support/have-i-got-breast-cancer/benign-breast-condi
tions/intraductal-papilloma.

"Breast: Other Benign Tumors; Intraductal Papilloma," Samuel
Bidot and Xiaoxian (Bill) Li for PathologyOutlines.com, Inc.,
last updated June 25, 2021, https://www.pathologyoutlines
.com/topic/breastpapilloma.html.

Latina breast cancer–patient support

Latinas Contra Cancer, http://latinascontracancer.org/

The Latino Cancer Institute, https://latinocancerinstitute.org/

LGBTQIA+ breast cancer–patient support

National LGBT Cancer Network, https://cancer-network.org/

National LGBT Cancer Project, https://www.lgbtcancer.org/

Lumpectomy

"Lumpectomy: The Procedure," Susan G. Komen (organization), Komen.org, updated May 18, 2021, https://www.komen.org/breast-cancer/treatment/type/surgery/lumpectomy/procedure-information/.

"Lumpectomy," Breastcancer.org, last modified March 9, 2019, https://www.breastcancer.org/treatment/surgery/lumpectomy.

"Meta-Analysis: Recurrence Rates after Lumpectomy Have Improved," Kristin Jenkins, News, *Medscape*, May 4, 2018, https://www.medscape.com/viewarticle/896185.

Lymph node biopsy: "Sentinel Lymph Node Biopsy," National Institutes of Health, National Cancer Institute, Cancer.gov, reviewed June 25, 2019, https://www.cancer.gov/about-cancer/diagnosis-staging/staging/sentinel-node-biopsy-fact-sheet.

MammaPrint, https://agendia.com

Mammography

"Mammography," RadiologyInfo.org, reviewed April 12, 2019, https://www.radiologyinfo.org/en/info.cfm?pg=mammo.

"Mammography: Everything You Need to Know about Your Mammogram," National Breast Cancer Foundation, Inc., accessed June 18, 2021, https://www.nationalbreastcancer.org/mammogram.

"Breast Cancer Screening Guidelines for Women," Centers for Disease Control and Prevention, CDC.gov, last reviewed September 22, 2020, https://www.cdc.gov/cancer/breast/pdf/breast-cancer-screening-guidelines-508.pdf.

"Mammograms," National Institutes of Health, National Cancer Institute, Cancer.gov, last reviewed December 7, 2016, https://www.cancer.gov/types/breast/mammograms-fact-sheet.

Mastectomy

"What Is Mastectomy?" Breastcancer.org, last modified October 29, 2020, https://www.breastcancer.org/treatment/surgery/mastectomy/what_is.

"Survival and Risk of Recurrence after Treatment," Susan G. Komen (organization), Komen.org, updated May 24, 2021, https://www.komen.org/breast-cancer/survivorship/medical-care/survival-and-risk-of-recurrence/.

Meditation and mindfulness for breast cancer patients

"Take a Moment with Meditation," American Cancer Society medical and editorial content team, Cancer.org, June 2, 2020, https://www.cancer.org/latest-news/take-a-moment-with-meditation.html.

"Meditation," Breastcancer.org, last modified May 5, 2020, https://www.breastcancer.org/treatment/comp_med/types/meditation.

Mental health: "Everything Is Awful and I'm Not Okay: Questions to Ask before Giving Up," University of Washington Family Medicine, 2015, https://depts.washington.edu/fammed/wp-content/uploads/2019/03/Katers-selfcare_printable.pdf

MRI: "Breast MRI," American Cancer Society medical and editorial content team, Cancer.org, last revised October 3, 2019, https://www.cancer.org/cancer/breast-cancer/screening-tests-and-early-detection/breast-mri-scans.html.

Native American/Indigenous/First Nations breast cancer–patient support: The American Indian Cancer Foundation, https://www.americanindiancancer.org/

Oncotype DX, https://www.oncotypeiq.com/en-US

Patient advocacy: "Breast Cancer Resource Directory," Patient Advocate Foundation, accessed June 25, 2021, https://www.patientadvocate.org/explore-our-resources/breast-cancer-resource-directory/.

PubMed database of peer-reviewed biomedical-science literature, https://pubmed.ncbi.nlm.nih.gov/

Radiation

Radiation Therapy and You: Support for People with Cancer, National Cancer Institute, NIH publication no. 17-7157 ([Washington, DC]: US Department of Heath and Human Services and the National Institutes of Health, 2016), https://www.cancer.gov/publications/patient-education/radiationttherapy.pdf.

"Radiation for Breast Cancer," American Cancer Society medical and editorial content team, Cancer.org, last revised September 19, 2019, https://www.cancer.org/cancer/breast-cancer/treatment/radiation-for-breast-cancer.html.

"Many Women Treated with Brachytherapy Aren't Good Candidates," Research News, Breastcancer.org, December 19, 2011, https://www.breastcancer.org/research-news/20111219.

Reconstruction

"Breast Reconstruction Surgery," American Cancer Society, Cancer.org, accessed June 25, 2021, https://www.cancer.org/cancer/breast-cancer/reconstruction-surgery.html.

"Breast Reconstruction," Breastcancer.org, last modified May 15, 2021, https://www.breastcancer.org/treatment/surgery/reconstruction.

Resensation study

"A New National Study Will Assess Microsurgery Reinnervation," Vanderbilt University Medical Center, Discover, July 3, 2019, https://discover.vumc.org/2019/07/resensation-after-breast-reconstruction/.

"Vanderbilt Surgeons Lead Nation in Study to Restore Sensation in Breast Tissue," Vanderbilt University Medical Center, VUMC Reporter, May 23, 2019, https://news.vumc.org/2019/05/23/vanderbilt-surgeons-lead-nation-in-study-to-restore-sensation-in-breast-tissue/.

"Revaree," Bonafide, accessed June 17, 2021, https://hello bonafide.com/products/revaree.

Scar management: "Caring for Scars after Breast Cancer Surgery," News and Personal Stories, Breast Cancer Now (website), March 8, 2017, https://breastcancernow.org/about-us/news-personal-stories/caring-scars-after-breast-cancer-surgery.

Surgery: "'If Ya Don't Know, Now Ya Know': A Guide to What Is Needed Post-mastectomy," Andy Sealy for Focus on Cancer Blog, Penn Medicine, Abramson Cancer Center, October 23, 2018, https://www.pennmedicine.org/cancer/about/focus-on-cancer/2018/october/list-of-post-mastectomy-items-needed.

Surgical drains

"Lumpectomy versus Mastectomy: I've Had 'Em Both and I'm Telling You All about It," Dana M. Brantley-Sieders, Talking Tatas, August 9, 2020. https://talkingtatas.com/2020/08/09/lumpectomy-versus-mastectomy-ive-had-em-both-and-im-telling-you-all-about-it/.

"Surgical Drains after Breast Surgery," Jean Campbell for Verywell Health, March 23, 2021, https://www.verywell health.com/managing-your-surgical-drains-following-breast -surgery-4021630.

Trans women and breast cancer risk: "Feminizing Hormones Linked to Higher Breast Cancer Risk in Trans Women, but Risk Still Lower than Average Woman's," Research News, Jamie De-Polo for Breastcancer.org, May 17, 2019, https://www.breast cancer.org/research-news/feminizing-hormones-increase-risk-in -trans-women.

Triple-negative breast cancer

"Triple-Negative Breast Cancer," Breastcancer.org, last modified April 9, 2021, https://www.breastcancer.org/symptoms/diagno-sis/trip_neg.

"Triple-Negative Breast Cancer," American Cancer Society med-ical and editorial content team, Cancer.org, last revised Janu-ary 27, 2021, https://www.cancer.org/cancer/breast-cancer/ understanding-a-breast-cancer-diagnosis/types-of-breast-can cer/triple-negative.html.

Trop-2-targeted therapy: "FDA News Release: FDA Approves New Therapy for Triple Negative Breast Cancer that Has Spread, Not Responded to Other Treatments," news release, US Food and Drug Administration, FDA.gov, April 22, 2020, https://www .fda.gov/news-events/press-announcements/fda-approves-new -therapy-triple-negative-breast-cancer-has-spread-not-re sponded-other-treatments.

Ultrasound: "Breast Ultrasound," Breast Imaging, Monica Pahuja for Inside Radiology (website), last modified August 13, 2018, https://www.insideradiology.com.au/breast-ultrasound/.

Vaccines

"Vaccine Types," Office of Infectious Diseases and HIV/AIDS Policy, HHS.gov, Vaccines.gov, April 29, 2021, https://www .vaccines.gov/basics/types.

"Breast Cancer Vaccine Shows Promise in Small Clinical Trial," Julia Evangelou Strait for the Siteman Cancer Center, Wash-ington University School of Medicine, accessed June 17, 2021, https://siteman.wustl.edu/breast-cancer-vaccine-shows -promise-in-small-clinical-trial/.

"Measles Virus-Based Immunovirotherapy in the Treatment of Metastatic Breast Cancer," Mayo Clinic Breast Cancer Spore, Mayo.edu, accessed June 17, 2021, https://www.mayo.edu/research/centers-programs/cancer-research/research-programs/womens-cancer-program/breast-cancer-spore/research-projects/measles-virus-based-immunovirotherapy-treatment-metastatic-breast-cancer.

"Vaginal Atrophy," Health Library, Cleveland Clinic, last reviewed October 27, 2020, https://my.clevelandclinic.org/health/diseases/15500-vaginal-atrophy.

Vaginal rejuvenation: "Urogenital Problems," Heather Currie, in collaboration with the medical advisory council of the British Menopause Society, Women's Health Concern (website), last reviewed August 2020, https://www.womens-health-concern.org/help-and-advice/factsheets/urogenital-problems/.

Women's Institute for Sexual Health, https://www.wishnashville.com/

Yoga with Adriene, https://www.youtube.com/user/yogawithadriene

~

Notes

Introduction

1. While one in eight cis women gets breast cancer, they aren't the only people who suffer from this disease. According to the CDC, one out of every one hundred breast cancers diagnosed in the United States is found in a man. Trans women and trans men can also be diagnosed with breast cancer (see chapter 6 for more on this), as can anyone of any gender identity who has mammary epithelial tissue in their body.

See Centers for Disease Control and Prevention, "Breast Cancer in Men," CDC.gov, last reviewed August 11, 2020, https://www.cdc.gov/cancer/breast/men/index.htm.

Chapter One

1. See, for example, Robert D. Cardiff and Sefton R. Wellings, "The Comparative Pathology of Human and Mouse Mammary Glands," *Journal of Mammary Gland Biology and Neoplasia* 4, no. 1 (January 1999): 105–22, https://doi.org/10.1023/a:1018712905244, https://www.ncbi.nlm.nih.gov/pubmed/10219910; and Robert D. Cardiff, Sonali Jindal, Piper M. Treuting, James J. Going, Barry Gusterson, and Henry J. Thompson, "Mammary Gland," in *Comparative Anatomy and Histology: A Mouse, Rat, and Human Atlas*, 2nd ed., ed. Piper M. Treuting, Suzanne M. Dintzis, and Kathleen S. Montine (London: Elsevier/Academic Press, 2018), 487–510.

2. See, for example, Robert D. Cardiff, "Validity of Mouse Mammary Tumour Models for Human Breast Cancer: Comparative Pathology," *Microscopy Research and Technique* 52, no. 2 (January 15 2001): 224–30, https://doi .org/10.1002/1097-0029(20010115)52:2<224::AID-JEMT1007>3.0.CO;2-A, https://www.ncbi.nlm.nih.gov/pubmed/11169869.

3. Check the video "Advances in Modeling Cancer in Mice: Technology, Biology, and Beyond," at the American Association for Cancer Research website, first presented at the AACR Conference on Advances on Modeling Cancer in Mice: Technology, Biology, and Beyond, Orlando, FL, September 24–27, 2017, https://www.aacr.org/blog/2017/09/21/how-mouse-models-pave -the-way-to-precision-cancer-medicine/.

4. Check these organizations out online at, respectively, https://olaw.nih .gov/home.htm, https://www.nih.gov/, and https://www.cancer.gov/.

5. For more information on IACUCs, visit https://www.aalas.org/iacuc.

6. They're online at https://www.aalas.org/.

7. For more on the benefits of using animals for medical testing, check out "Medical Benefits," Speaking of Research (website), accessed June 18, 2021, https://speakingofresearch.com/facts/medical-benefits/.

Chapter Two

1. Siddhartha Mukherjee, *The Emperor of All Maladies: A Biography of Cancer* (New York: Scribner, 2010).

2. They're online at https://cdmrp.army.mil/.

3. Edward J. Odes et al., "Earliest Hominin Cancer: 1.7-Million-Year-Old Osteosarcoma from Swartkrans Cave, South Africa," research article, *South African Journal of Science* 112, nos. 7/8 (2016): 1–5, https://doi.org/ https://doi.org/10.17159/sajs.2016/20150471, http://www.scielo.org.za/scielo .php?pid=S0038-23532016000400014&script=sci_arttext&tlng=es.

4. See, for example, Douglas Hanahan and Robert A. Weinberg, "Hallmarks of Cancer: The Next Generation," *Cell* 144, no. 5 (March 4, 2011): 646–74, https://doi.org/10.1016/j.cell.2011.02.013, https://www.ncbi.nlm.nih .gov/pubmed/21376230.

5. CancerQuest—a nonprofit educational initiative of Emory University's Winship Cancer Institute—has a great video on the subject, at "Animated Introduction to Cancer Biology (Full Documentary)," accessed June 18, 2021, http://www.cancerquest.org/patients/what-cancer.

6. For a beautiful illustration of this concept, see RIKEN Omics Science Center's video "The Central Dogma: From Genomic Information to Protein Synthesis," made as part of the Beyond Genetics exhibit at the National Sci-

ence Museum of Japan, 2007, https://www.youtube.com/watch?v=-ygpqVr7_xs.

7. For more information, check out "BRCA: The Breast Cancer Gene," National Breast Cancer Foundation, Inc. (website), medically reviewed April 15, 2020, https://www.nationalbreastcancer.org/what-is-brca.

8. I cover this in my blog; see Dana M. Brantley-Sieders, "Science Break! Outreach: Getting High School Students Excited about Cancer Research," *Talking Tatas*, January 20, 2020, https://talkingtatas.com/2020/01/20/science-break-outreach-getting-high-school-students-excited-about-cancer-research/.

9. This video by the *SciShow* explains this concept beautifully and with lots of great visuals: "Why We Haven't Cured Cancer," uploaded May 14, 2015, https://www.youtube.com/watch?v=7tzaWOdvGMw.

10. "Types," National Breast Cancer Foundation, Inc. (website), medically reviewed April 15, 2020, https://www.nationalbreastcancer.org/types-of-breast-cancer/.

11. More on that in chapter 3; and see table 2.1 for more information on this classification system.

12. "Cancer Stat Facts: Female Breast Cancer Subtypes," National Cancer Institute, Surveillance, Epidemiology, and End Results Program, accessed June 25, 2021, https://seer.cancer.gov/statfacts/html/breast-subtypes.html.

13. David R. Hout, "A Disease with Many Faces," Diagnostics, *The Pathologist*, May 3, 2019, https://thepathologist.com/diagnostics/a-disease-with-many-faces.

14. For an excellent overview of cancer as an evolutionary process, see Yale Courses' video "Cancer as an Evolutionary Process: Clonal Evolution," uploaded May 14, 2014, https://www.youtube.com/watch?v=wH9jmQglOLw.

15. The National Cancer Institute has produced a video providing an excellent overview of this process: "Metastasis: How Cancer Spreads," National Cancer Institute, National Institutes of Health, US Department of Health and Human Services, December 2016, https://www.youtube.com/watch?v=fQwar_-QdiQ.

Chapter Three

1. According to the National Institutes of Health, 284,200 new cases of breast cancer will be diagnosed in 2021. See American Cancer Society, "Estimates for 2021," Cancer Statistics Center, Cancer.org, accessed July 15, 2021, https://cancerstatisticscenter.cancer.org/?_ga=2.27173118.2100259821.1626382499-2110999834.1626382499#!/.

2. For more information and a visual explanation of mammography, visit RadiologyInfo.org online at "Mammography," https://www.radiologyinfo.org/ en/info.cfm?pg=mammo (reviewed April 12, 2019). And for "Everything You Need to Know about Your Mammogram," visit the National Breast Cancer Foundation, Inc., at https://www.nationalbreastcancer.org/mammogram (accessed June 18, 2021); their site also offers information on breast self-exams and clinical exams.

3. "Breast Cancer Screening Guidelines for Women," Centers for Disease Control and Prevention, CDC.gov, last reviewed September 22, 2020, https:// www.cdc.gov/cancer/breast/pdf/breast-cancer-screening-guidelines-508.pdf.

4. For more on this, check out the CDC's list at "What Are the Risk Factors for Breast Cancer?" CDC.gov, last reviewed September 14, 2020, https://www .cdc.gov/cancer/breast/basic_info/risk_factors.htm.

5. Learn how at "Breast Self-Exam," Breastcancer.org, last modified October 24, 2019, https://www.breastcancer.org/symptoms/testing/types/self_exam.

6. Learn more at "Mammograms," National Institutes of Health, National Cancer Institute, Cancer.gov, last reviewed December 7, 2016, https://www .cancer.gov/types/breast/mammograms-fact-sheet.

7. For more information on breast MRI, check out the American Cancer Society's article on "Breast MRI," written by the AMC's medical and editorial content team, Cancer.org, last revised October 3, 2019, https://www.cancer .org/cancer/breast-cancer/screening-tests-and-early-detection/breast-mri-scans .html.

8. For more information, check out Monica Pahuja, "Breast Ultrasound," Breast Imaging, Inside Radiology (website), last modified August 13, 2018, https://www.insideradiology.com.au/breast-ultrasound/.

9. Wendie A. Berg et al., "Cancer Yield and Patterns of Follow-Up for BI-RADS Category 3 after Screening Mammography Recall in the National Mammography Database," *Radiology* 296, no. 1 (July 2020): 32–41, https://doi.org/10.1148/radiol.2020192641, https://www.ncbi.nlm.nih.gov/ pubmed/32427557.

Chapter Four

1. Learn more about Oncotype DX at https://www.oncotypeiq.com/en-US.

2. See "Hereditary Breast Cancer and BRCA Genes," Centers for Disease Control and Prevention, CDC.gov, last reviewed April 5, 2019, https://www .cdc.gov/cancer/breast/young_women/bringyourbrave/hereditary_breast_can cer/.

3. See Sarah M. Bernhardt et al., "Hormonal Modulation of Breast Cancer Gene Expression: Implications for Intrinsic Subtyping in Premenopausal Women," *Frontiers in Oncology* 6 (November 2016): 241, https://doi.org/10.3389/fonc.2016.00241, https://www.ncbi.nlm.nih.gov/pubmed/27896218; and see Andrea Nicolini, Paola Ferrari, and Michael J. Duffy, "Prognostic and Predictive Biomarkers in Breast Cancer: Past, Present and Future," *Seminars in Cancer Biology* 52, part 1 (October 2018): 56–73, https://doi.org/10.1016/j.semcancer.2017.08.010; https://www.ncbi.nlm.nih.gov/pubmed/28882552.

4. See Katya Losk et al., "Oncotype DX Testing in Early-Stage Node-Positive Breast Cancer and Impact on Chemotherapy Use at a Comprehensive Cancer Center," Abstract, *Journal of Clinical Oncology* 37, 15, supplement (2019): 549, https://doi.org/10.1200/JCO.2019.37.15_suppl.549, https://ascopubs.org/doi/abs/10.1200/JCO.2019.37.15_suppl.549.

5. This is both frightening and liberating. New information from ongoing studies is changing the interpretation of studies and recommendations all the time. The standard of care today might be very different from what is considered standard of care ten to twenty years from now. Had I been diagnosed five to ten years earlier than 2018, my standard of care would most likely have included chemo.

6. Learn more about the MammaPrint at https://agendia.com/.

7. For a list of genes in the MammaPrint test, see Sun Tian et al., "Biological Functions of the Genes in the MammaPrint Breast Cancer Profile Reflect the Hallmarks of Cancer," *Biomarker Insights* 5 (November 28, 2010): 129–38, https://doi.org/10.4137/BMI.S6184, https://www.ncbi.nlm.nih.gov/pubmed/21151591.

8. Visit them online at https://www.foundationmedicine.com/.

9. "FDA Clears World's First and Only Wire-Free Radar Breast Tumor Localization System for Long Term Implant Capabilities," news release, Cianna Medical Group, November 13, 2017, https://www.ciannamedical.com/cianna_news_releases/fda-clears-worlds-first-wire-free-radar-breast-tumor-localization-system-long-term-implant-capabilities/ (link inactive), text available at https://www.globenewswire.com/en/news-release/2017/11/13/1185036/37185/en/FDA-Clears-World-s-First-and-Only-Wire-Free-Radar-Breast-Tumor-Localization-System-for-Long-Term-Implant-Capabilities.html.

10. Learn more about the procedure at "Lumpectomy: The Procedure," Susan G. Komen (organization), Komen.org, updated May 18, 2021, https://www.komen.org/breast-cancer/treatment/type/surgery/lumpectomy/procedure-information/.

11. Dana M. Brantley-Sieders, "Lumpectomy versus Mastectomy: I've Had 'Em Both and I'm Telling You All about It," *Talking Tatas*, August 9, 2020, https://talkingtatas.com/2020/08/09/lumpectomy-versus-mastectomy-ive-had -em-both-and-im-telling-you-all-about-it/.

12. BTW, if you aren't familiar with Tig Notaro's work, treat yourself! She talks about her experience with breast cancer in her album *Live* and shows off her beautiful, flat chest in her HBO special, *Boyish Girl Interrupted*. The first time I laughed after my diagnosis was listening to *Live*. Tig Notaro, *Live*, album, Pig Newton (label), released October 5, 2012; Tig Notaro, *Boyish Girl Interrupted*, album, Bentzen Ball Records and Secretly Canadian (labels), released August 5, 2016, and streaming on HBO at https://www.hbo.com/ specials/tig-notaro-boyish-girl-interrupted/synopsis.

13. For example, *Breast Cancer Straight Talk*, a private group on Facebook, at https://www.facebook.com/groups/Straighttalkbreastcancersupport/.

14. Visit these organizations online at, respectively, https://reach.cancer. org/, https://www.breastcancer.org/treatment/comp_med/types/group, https:// www.nationalbreastcancer.org/nbcf-programs/breast-cancer-support-group, and https://www.cancersupportcommunity.org/.

15. "A New National Study Will Assess Microsurgery Reinnervation," *Discover*, Vanderbilt University Medical Center, July 3, 2019, https://discover .vumc.org/2019/07/resensation-after-breast-reconstruction/.

16. "Vanderbilt Surgeons Lead Nation in Study to Restore Sensation in Breast Tissue," *VUMC Reporter*, Vanderbilt University Medical Center, May 23, 2019, https://news.vumc.org/2019/05/23/vanderbilt-surgeons-lead-nation -in-study-to-restore-sensation-in-breast-tissue/.

17. See Kristin Jenkins, "Meta-Analysis: Recurrence Rates after Lumpec- tomy Have Improved," News, *Medscape*, May 4, 2018, https://www.medscape .com/viewarticle/896185; and see Heather Neuman et al., "Local Recurrence Rates after Breast-Conserving Therapy in Patients Receiving Modern Era Therapy," American Society of Breast Surgeons, nineteenth annual meeting, Orlando, FL, May 4, 2018, and see pp. 19–20 in https://www.breastsurgeons .org/docs/resources/old_meetings/2018_Official_Proceedings_ASBrS.pdf.

18. See Jay R. Harris and Monica Morrow, "Breast-Conserving Therapy," in *Diseases of the Breast*, 5th ed., ed. Jay R. Harris, Marc E. Lippman, Monica Morrow, and C. Kent Osborne (Philadelphia: Wolters Kluwer Health, 2014), 514–35; and see "Survival and Risk of Recurrence after Treatment," Susan G. Komen (organization), Komen.org, updated May 24, 2021, https://www .komen.org/breast-cancer/survivorship/medical-care/survival-and-risk-of-re currence/.

19. See Jon Johnson, "Depression after Surgery: What You Need to Know," *Medical News Today*, August 20, 2019, https://www.medicalnewstoday.com/articles/317616.

20. The University of Pennsylvania has some great information about essentials for surgery and recovery, and check out Breast Cancer Now's helpful tips for scar management: Andy Sealy, "'If Ya Don't Know, Now Ya Know': A Guide to What Is Needed Post-mastectomy," *Focus on Cancer Blog*, Penn Medicine, Abramson Cancer Center, October 23, 2018, https://www.pennmedicine.org/cancer/about/focus-on-cancer/2018/october/list-of-post-mastectomy-items-needed; and see "Caring for Scars after Breast Cancer Surgery," News and Personal Stories. Breast Cancer Now (website), March 8, 2017, https://breastcancernow.org/about-us/news-personal-stories/caring-scars-after-breast-cancer-surgery.

And for more information on surgery and breast reconstruction—from implants and autologous to flat or one-breasted, including personal stories and some beautiful photographs of survivors, check out Patricia Anstett, *Breast Cancer Surgery and Reconstruction: What's Right for You*, photog. Kathleen Galligan (Lanham, MD: Rowman & Littlefield, 2016).

Chapter Five

1. For more information on this treatment, see National Cancer Institute, *Radiation Therapy and You: Support for People with Cancer*, NIH publication no. 17-7157 ([Washington, DC]: US Department of Heath and Human Services and the National Institutes of Health, 2016), https://www.cancer.gov/publications/patient-education/radiationttherapy.pdf.

2. For more on this program, visit https://www.komen.org/wp-content/uploads/2020-Komen-TAP-Helpline-Flyer-Eng-Aug-2.pdf; and contact the Komen Breast Care Helpline directly at 1-877-GO-KOMEN, or 1-877-465-6636.

3. "Financial Assistance," Susan G. Komen, accessed June 17, 2021, https://www.komen.org/support-resources/financial-assistance/financial-assistance-options/.

4. Visit these organizations online at, respectively, at https://www.cancercare.org/questions/136, https://www.pinkfund.org/, http://mbcn.org/finding-financial-assistance/, https://www.lbbc.org/get-support/additional-resources, and https://www.abcf.org/programs/breast-cancer-assistance-program.

5. See "Radiation for Breast Cancer," American Cancer Society, Cancer.org, last revised September 19, 2019, https://www.cancer.org/cancer/breast-cancer/treatment/radiation-for-breast-cancer.html; and "Many Women

Treated with Brachytherapy Aren't Good Candidates," Research News, Breastcancer.org, December 19, 2011, https://www.breastcancer.org/research -news/20111219.

6. For more information, see the National Cancer Institute, *Chemotherapy and You: Support for People with Cancer*, NIH publication no. 18-7157 ([Washington, DC]: US Department of Health and Human Services and the National Cancer Institute Office of Communications and Public Liaison, 2018), https:// www.cancer.gov/publications/patient-education/chemotherapy-and-you.pdf.

7. For more on this kind of breast cancer treatment, see "How Is Chemotherapy Given?" Breastcancer.org, last modified March 25, 2020, https://www .breastcancer.org/treatment/chemotherapy/process/how.

8. See Mayo Clinic staff, "Chemotherapy for Breast Cancer," MayoClinic. org, February 24, 2021, https://www.mayoclinic.org/tests-procedures/chemo therapy-for-breast-cancer/about/pac-20384931.

9. See American Cancer Society medical and editorial content team, "Chemo Brain," American Cancer Society, Cancer.org, last revised February 1, 2020, https://www.cancer.org/treatment/treatments-and-side-effects/ physical-side-effects/changes-in-mood-or-thinking/chemo-brain.html.

10. Check out her YouTube channel at https://www.youtube.com/user/ yogawithadriene.

11. "Everything Is Awful and I'm Not Okay: Questions to Ask before Giving Up," University of Washington Family Medicine, 2015, https://depts. washington.edu/fammed/wp-content/uploads/2019/03/Katers-selfcare_print able.pdf.

12. Or maybe they did. In which case, you're welcome, my neighbors.

13. See "How to Read Hormone Receptor Test Results," Breastcancer.org, last modified September 21, 2020, https://www.breastcancer.org/symptoms/ diagnosis/hormone_status/read_results.

14. See "Lupron Depot® 7.5 Mg (Leuprolide Acetate for Depot Suspension)," drug information sheet, US Food and Drug Administration, FDA.gov, October 7, 2011, https://www.accessdata.fda.gov/drugsatfda_docs/ label/2012/019732s038lbl.pdf.

15. Read more about the ELAINE trial at "Evaluation of Lasofoxifene versus Fulvestrant in Advanced or Metastatic ER+/HER2− Breast Cancer with an ESR1 Mutation," ClinicalTrials.gov, US National Library of Medicine, National Institutes of Health, accessed June 18, 2021, https://clinicaltrials.gov/ ct2/show/NCT03781063.

16. See American Cancer Society medical and editorial content team, "Hormone Therapy for Breast Cancer," American Cancer Society, Cancer.org,

last revised September 18, 2019, https://www.cancer.org/cancer/breast-cancer/ treatment/hormone-therapy-for-breast-cancer.html.

17. Ed. Ann Godoff (New York: Random House, 2011).

18. See "HER2+ Breast Cancer Survival Rates," Breast Cancer Guide, WebMD, last reviewed May 17, 2020, https://www.webmd.com/breast-cancer/ guide/her2-positive-breast-cancer-survival-rates.

19. See "Herceptin Dosing and Administration," Herceptin.com, accessed March 15, 2021, https://www.herceptin.com/hcp/dosing-admin.html.

20. See "DMC Has Concluded that OlympiA Trial of Lynparza Crossed Superiority Boundary for Invasive Disease-Free Survival vs. Placebo at Planned Interim Analysis," news release, AstraZeneca, February 17, 2021, https://www .astrazeneca.com/media-centre/press-releases/2021/olympia-trial-of-lynparza -idmc-recommend-early-analysis.html.

21. See "FDA News Release: FDA Approves New Therapy for Triple Negative Breast Cancer that Has Spread, Not Responded to Other Treatments," news release, US Food and Drug Administration, FDA.gov, April 22, 2020, https://www.fda.gov/news-events/press-announcements/fda-approves -new-therapy-triple-negative-breast-cancer-has-spread-not-responded-other -treatments.

22. For more on these risks and options related to childbearing after cancer treatments (e.g., harvesting and freezing eggs prior to treatment, harvesting and freezing ovarian tissue, egg donors, in vitro fertilization, surrogacy, and so on), see "Fertility Issues," Breastcancer.org, last modified July 22, 2020, https:// www.breastcancer.org/treatment/side_effects/fertility_issues.

23. Lesbian, gay, bisexual, transgender, queer, questioning, intersex, and asexual folks, plus other identities on the spectrum of sexuality and gender identity.

Chapter Six

1. The organization, which has since shortened its name, was then known as Susan G. Komen for the Cure.

2. Check them out online at https://seer.cancer.gov.

3. Read about our analysis at Dana M. Brantley-Sieders et al., "Local Breast Cancer Spatial Patterning: A Tool for Community Health Resource Allocation to Address Local Disparities in Breast Cancer Mortality," *PLoS One* 7, no. 9 (September 2012): e45238, https://doi.org/10.1371/journal.pone.0045238, https://www.ncbi.nlm.nih.gov/pubmed/23028869.

4. Read more about it at Lisa A. Newman and Linda M. Kaljee, "Health Disparities and Triple-Negative Breast Cancer in African American Women: A Review," *JAMA Surgery* 152, no. 5 (May 1, 2017): 485–93, https://doi.org/10.1001/jamasurg.2017.0005, https://www.ncbi.nlm.nih.gov/pubmed/28355428.

5. Gina Martinez, "GoFundMe CEO: One-Third of Site's Donations Are to Cover Medical Costs," US, Healthcare, *Time*, updated January 30, 2019, https://time.com/5516037/gofundme-medical-bills-one-third-ceo/.

6. K. Robin Yabroff et al., "Health Insurance Coverage Disruptions and Cancer Care and Outcomes: Systematic Review of Published Research," *Journal of the National Cancer Institute* 112, no. 7 (July 1, 2020): 671–87, https://doi.org/10.1093/jnci/djaa048, https://www.ncbi.nlm.nih.gov/pubmed/32337585.

7. Christine D. Hsu et al., "Breast Cancer Stage Variation and Survival in Association with Insurance Status and Sociodemographic Factors in US Women 18 to 64 Years Old," *Cancer* 123, no. 16 (August 15, 2017): 3125–31, https://doi.org/10.1002/cncr.30722, https://www.ncbi.nlm.nih.gov/pubmed/28440864.

8. K. Robin Yabroff et al., "Minimizing the Burden of Cancer in the United States: Goals for a High-Performing Health Care System," *CA: A Cancer Journal for Clinicians* 69, no. 3 (May/June 2019): 170 and throughout, https://doi.org/10.3322/caac.21556, https://www.ncbi.nlm.nih.gov/pubmed/30786025.

9. Hsu et al., "Breast Cancer Stage Variation."

10. Liam Davenport, "Is There an Ideal Healthcare System for Treating Cancer?" *Medscape Oncology*, September 24, 2019, https://www.medscape.com/viewarticle/918795#vp_2.

11. Ahmedin Jemal et al., "Factors that Contributed to Black-White Disparities in Survival among Nonelderly Women with Breast Cancer between 2004 and 2013," *Journal of Clinical Oncology* 36, no. 1 (January 1, 2018): 14–24, https://doi.org/10.1200/JCO.2017.73.7932, https://www.ncbi.nlm.nih.gov/pubmed/29035645.

12. Maria Aspan, "'We Can't Ever Go to the Doctor without Our Guard Down': Why Black Women Are 40% More Likely to Die of Breast Cancer," *Fortune*, June 30, 2020, https://fortune.com/2020/06/30/black-women-breast-cancer-mortality-racism-healthcare-pandemic/.

13. Tina K. Sacks, *Invisible Visits: Black Middle-Class Women in the American Healthcare System* (Oxford: Oxford University Press, 2019).

14. Louis A. Penner et al., "An Analysis of Race-Related Attitudes and Beliefs in Black Cancer Patients: Implications for Health Care Disparities," *Journal of Health Care for the Poor and Underserved* 27, no. 3 (2016): 1503–20, https://doi.org/10.1353/hpu.2016.0115, https://www.ncbi.nlm.nih.gov/

pubmed/27524781; Darcell P. Scharff et al., "More than Tuskegee: Understanding Mistrust about Research Participation," *Journal of Health Care for the Poor and Underserved* 21, no. 3 (August 2010): 879–97, https://doi.org/10.1353/hpu.0.0323, https://www.ncbi.nlm.nih.gov/pubmed/20693733.

15. Deirdre Cooper Owens, *Medical Bondage: Race, Gender, and the Origins of American Gynecology* (Athens: University of Georgia Press, 2018).

16. DeNeen L. Brown, "'You've Got Bad Blood': The Horror of the Tuskegee Syphilis Experiment," Retropolis, *Washington Post*, May 16, 2017, https://www.washingtonpost.com/news/retropolis/wp/2017/05/16/youve-got-bad-blood-the-horror-of-the-tuskegee-syphilis-experiment/.

17. Rebecca Skloot, *The Immortal Life of Henrietta Lacks* (New York: Crown Publishing Group, 2010).

18. April Dembosky, "Stop Blaming Tuskegee, Critics Say. It's Not an 'Excuse' for Current Medical Racism," NPR.org, March 23, 2021, https://www.npr.org/sections/health-shots/2021/03/23/974059870/stop-blaming-tuskegee-critics-say-its-not-an-excuse-for-current-medical-racism.

19. Janice A. Sabin, "How We Fail Black Patients in Pain.," Insights, *Association of American Medical Colleges News*, January 6, 2020, https://www.aamc.org/news-insights/how-we-fail-black-patients-pain; and see Wanda Sykes, *Wanda Sykes: Not Normal*, Netflix, released May 21, 2019, https://www.netflix.com/title/81011598.

20. Valentina A. Zavala et al., "Cancer Health Disparities in Racial/Ethnic Minorities in the United States," *British Journal of Cancer* 124, no. 2 (January 2021): 315–32, https://doi.org/10.1038/s41416-020-01038-6, https://www.ncbi.nlm.nih.gov/pubmed/32901135.

21. Giorgio Sirugo, Scott M. Williams, and Sarah A. Tishkoff, "The Missing Diversity in Human Genetic Studies," *Cell* 177, no. 4 (May 2, 2019): 1080, https://doi.org/10.1016/j.cell.2019.04.032, https://pubmed.ncbi.nlm.nih.gov/31051100/.

22. Reviewed in Zavala et al., "Cancer Health Disparities."

23. Ulrike Boehmer, "LGBT Populations' Barriers to Cancer Care," *Seminars in Oncology Nursing* 34, no. 1 (February 2018): 21–29, https://doi.org/10.1016/j.soncn.2017.11.002, https://www.ncbi.nlm.nih.gov/pubmed/29338894.

24. "Cancer Disparities," National Institutes of Health, National Cancer Institute, Cancer.gov, updated November 17, 2020, https://www.cancer.gov/about-cancer/understanding/disparities.

25. Boehmer, "LGBT Populations' Barriers."

26. Mandi L. Pratt-Chapman and Jennifer Potter, *Cancer Care Considerations for Sexual and Gender Minority Patients* ([Rockville, MD]: Association of Community Cancer Centers, 2019), https://www.accc-cancer.org/docs/

documents/oncology-issues/articles/nd19/nd19-cancer-care-considerations
-for-sexual-and-gender-minority-patients.pdf.

27. Boehmer, "LGBT Populations' Barriers."

28. "Hormones," National Institutes of Health, National Cancer Institute, Cancer.gov, April 29, 2015, https://www.cancer.gov/about-cancer/causes
-prevention/risk/hormones.

29. "Using HRT (Hormone Replacement Therapy)," Breastcancer.org, last modified April 21, 2021, https://www.breastcancer.org/risk/factors/hrt.

30. Christel J. M. de Blok et al., "Breast Cancer Risk in Transgender People Receiving Hormone Treatment: Nationwide Cohort Study in the Netherlands," BMJ 365 (May 14, 2019): 11652, https://doi.org/10.1136/bmj.11652, https://www.ncbi.nlm.nih.gov/pubmed/31088823.

31. The findings of this study are also summarized in Jamie DePolo, "Feminizing Hormones Linked to Higher Breast Cancer Risk in Trans Women, but Risk Still Lower than Average Woman's," Research News, Breastcancer.org, May 17, 2019, https://www.breastcancer.org/research-news/feminizing
-hormones-increase-risk-in-trans-women.

32. Lisa I. Iezzoni et al., "Associations between Disability and Breast or Cervical Cancers, Accounting for Screening Disparities," Medical Care 59, no. 2 (February 1, 2021): 139–47, https://doi.org/10.1097/MLR.0000000000001449, https://www.ncbi.nlm.nih.gov/pubmed/33201087.

33. C. Brooke Steele et al., "Prevalence of Cancer Screening among Adults with Disabilities, United States, 2013," Preventing Chronic Disease 14 (January 26, 2017): E09, https://doi.org/10.5888/pcd14.160312, https://www.ncbi.nlm
.nih.gov/pubmed/28125399.

34. Rochelle Strenger, Howard Safran, and Cooper Woodward, "Autism and Cancer: Creating Comprehensive Solutions for Complex Needs," ASCO Daily News, January 3, 2020, https://dailynews.ascopubs.org/do/10.1200/
ADN.19.190488/full/.

35. Laurie Margolies and Shivani Chaudhry, "Pushing Anxiety as a Risk of Screening Mammography Is Benevolent Sexism and Bad for Women's Health Outcomes," Clinical Imaging 68 (December 2020): 166–68, https://
doi.org/10.1016/j.clinimag.2020.05.034, https://www.ncbi.nlm.nih.gov/
pubmed/32645603.

36. Margolies and Chaudhry, "Pushing Anxiety as a Risk."

37. For more resources in finding advocacy in better care, visit https://www
.patientadvocate.org/explore-our-resources/breast-cancer-resource-directory/.

38. Sana Goldberg, How to Be a Patient: The Essential Guide to Navigating the World of Modern Medicine (New York: HarperCollins, 2019).

39. Catherine Guthrie, "These Cancer Patients Wanted to Get Rid of Their Breasts for Good. Their Doctors Had Other Ideas," *Cosmopolitan*, September 6, 2018, https://www.cosmopolitan.com/health-fitness/a22984204/breast-cancer-survivors-mastectomy-sexism/.

40. Check out Kim Bowles's initiative at https://notputtingonashirt.org/.

41. "Reducing Disparities in Health Care," Patient Support and Advocacy, American Medical Association, accessed June 17, 2021, https://www.ama-assn.org/delivering-care/patient-support-advocacy/reducing-disparities-health-care.

42. Donita C. Brady and Ashanti T. Weeraratna, "The Race toward Equity: Increasing Racial Diversity in Cancer Research and Cancer Care," *Cancer Discovery* 10, no. 10 (Oct 2020): 1451–54, https://doi.org/10.1158/2159-8290.CD-20-1193, https://www.ncbi.nlm.nih.gov/pubmed/32816861.

43. "Cultural Competence Training for Health Care Professionals," County Health Rankings (website), University of Wisconsin Population Health Institute, last updated January 17, 2020, https://www.countyhealthrankings.org/take-action-to-improve-health/what-works-for-health/strategies/cultural-competence-training-for-health-care-professionals.

44. American Association for Cancer Research, *AACR Cancer Disparities Progress Report 2020: Achieving the Bold Vision of Health Equity for Racial and Ethnic Minorities and Other Underserved Populations* (Philadelphia: American Association for Cancer Research, 2020), http://www.CancerDisparitiesProgressReport.org/ and https://cancerprogressreport.aacr.org/wp-content/uploads/sites/2/2020/09/AACR_CDPR_2020.pdf.

45. Visit each of these organizations online at, respectively, https://www.nih.gov/, https://www.cancer.gov/, and https://www.cancer.gov/about-nci/organization/crchd/disparities-research/basic-research.

46. Brady and Weeraratna, "The Race toward Equity."

47. Find out more about them at https://www.blackincancer.com/.

48. American Association for Cancer Research, *AACR Cancer Disparities Progress Report 2020: Achieving the Bold Vision of Health Equity for Racial and Ethnic Minorities and Other Underserved Populations* (Philadelphia: American Association for Cancer Research, 2020), http://www.CancerDisparitiesProgressReport.org/ and https://cancerprogressreport.aacr.org/wp-content/uploads/sites/2/2020/09/AACR_CDPR_2020.pdf.

49. Check them out online at, respectively, https://www.aacr.org/ and https://www.cancer.org/.

Chapter Seven

1. *Really* want to get that put on a business card.

2. Check out *The Immortal Life of Henrietta Lacks* by Rebecca Skloot for the astounding tale of how one woman's cancer cells were harvested without her knowledge or permission and have since become crucial to cancer-treatment research.

3. Read more at "Fibroadenoma," American Society of Breast Surgeons, Breast360.org, accessed June 17, 2021, https://breast360.org/topic/2015/10/24/fibroadenoma/.

4. Read more at "Intraductal Papilloma," Breast Cancer Now (website), last reviewed December 2018, https://breastcancernow.org/information-support/have-i-got-breast-cancer/benign-breast-conditions/intraductal-papilloma.

5. Find out more at American Cancer Society, *Cancer Facts and Figures, 2020* (Atlanta: American Cancer Society, 2020), https://www.cancer.org/content/dam/cancer-org/research/cancer-facts-and-statistics/annual-cancer-facts-and-figures/2020/cancer-facts-and-figures-2020.pdf.

6. And see American Cancer Society, *Breast Cancer Facts and Figures, 2019–2020* (Atlanta: American Cancer Society, Inc., 2019), https://www.cancer.org/content/dam/cancer-org/research/cancer-facts-and-statistics/breast-cancer-facts-and-figures/breast-cancer-facts-and-figures-2019-2020.pdf.

Chapter Eight

1. Visit Gilda's Club online at https://www.cancersupportcommunity.org/mission-vision-and-history.

2. Find out more at "What Is Cognitive Behavioral Therapy?" American Psychological Association, APA.org, July 2017, https://www.apa.org/ptsd-guideline/patients-and-families/cognitive-behavioral.

3. *Cancer Health* staff, "Finding Inspiration in Patton Oswalt's 'It's Chaos. Be Kind,'" *Cancer Health* blog, November 10, 2017, https://www.cancerhealth.com/blog/finding-inspiration-in-patton-oswalt-its-chaos-be-kind. And see Patton Oswalt, *Patton Oswalt: Annihilation*, Netflix, released October 17, 2017, https://www.netflix.com/title/80177406.

4. American Cancer Society medical and editorial content team, "Take a Moment with Meditation," American Cancer Society, Cancer.org, June 2, 2020, https://www.cancer.org/latest-news/take-a-moment-with-meditation.html.

Chapter Nine

1. Refer back to chapter 4, note 10, for an explanation of SAVI SCOUT technology.

2. (I don't know if there are any new *Saw* movies planned, but if so, this would make one hell of a trap.)

3. At this point, I know she's either doing dishes or pouring a glass of wine. I hope it's wine.

4. I have the *best* friends.

5. Though arguably mentally as well?

6. At least he was kind enough not to film me.

7. Jim Ridley, "Losing the Connection," *Nashville Scene*, March 17, 2005, https://www.nashvillescene.com/news/article/13011506/losing-the-connection.

8. The QIA+ would come later.

9. The pervasive homophobia of the day resulted in at least one horrific hate crime that ended the life of an area man. Sue Ann Pressley, "Hate May Have Triggered Fatal Barracks Beating," *Washington Post*, August 11, 1999, https://www.washingtonpost.com/wp-srv/national/daily/aug99/winchell11.htm.

10. It's like he hates fun.

Chapter Ten

1. See, for example, "Meditation," Breastcancer.org, last modified May 5, 2020, https://www.breastcancer.org/treatment/comp_med/types/meditation.

2. Erin Blakemore, "1,800 Studies Later, Scientists Conclude Homeopathy Doesn't Work," Smart News, *Smithsonian Magazine*, March 11, 2015, https://www.smithsonianmag.com/smart-news/1800-studies-later-scientists-conclude-homeopathy-doesnt-work-180954534/.

3. "How Does Complementary Medicine Work?" Breastcancer.org, last modified May 5, 2020, https://www.breastcancer.org/treatment/comp_med/what_is_it/how_it_works.

4. Skyler B. Johnson et al., "Complementary Medicine, Refusal of Conventional Cancer Therapy, and Survival among Patients with Curable Cancers," *JAMA Oncology* 4, no. 10 (October 1, 2018): 1375–81, https://doi.org/10.1001/jamaoncol.2018.2487, https://www.ncbi.nlm.nih.gov/pubmed/30027204.

5. Marian L. Neuhouser et al., "Use of Complementary and Alternative Medicine and Breast Cancer Survival in the Health, Eating, Activity, and Lifestyle Study," *Breast Cancer Research and Treatment* 160, no. 3 (December 2016): 539–46, https://doi.org/10.1007/s10549-016-4010-x, https://www.ncbi.nlm.nih.gov/pubmed/27766453.

6. You can find my blog, *Talking Tatas*, at https://talkingtatas.com/.

7. Skyler B. Johnson et al., "Use of Alternative Medicine for Cancer and Its Impact on Survival," *Journal of the National Cancer Institute* 110, no. 1 (January 1, 2018), https://doi.org/10.1093/jnci/djx145, https://www.ncbi.nlm.nih.gov/pubmed/28922780.

8. Jillian Kubala, "7 Uses and Benefits of CBD Oil (Plus Side Effects)," *Healthline*, February 26, 2018, https://www.healthline.com/nutrition/cbd-oil-benefits.

9. Read more at PDQ® Integrative, Alternative, and Complementary Therapies Editorial Board, *PDQ Cannabis and Cannabinoids* (Bethesda, MD: National Cancer Institute, updated June 3, 2021), https://www.cancer.gov/about-cancer/treatment/cam/hp/cannabis-pdq.

10. See Siyu Shi et al., "False News of a Cannabis Cancer Cure," *Cureus* 11, no. 1 (January 19, 2019): e3918, https://doi.org/10.7759/cureus.3918, https://www.ncbi.nlm.nih.gov/pubmed/30931189.

11. Mike Adams, "Science Tells Us Marijuana Doesn't Kill Cancer, So Does Real Life," *Forbes*, October 8, 2018, https://www.forbes.com/sites/mikeadams/2018/10/08/science-tells-us-marijuana-doesnt-kill-cancer-so-does-real-life.

12. Read more about the study at "Effects of Cannabis Use in Stage III–IV Non-small Cell Lung Cancer Patients," National Institutes of Health, National Cancer Institute, Cancer.gov, accessed June 24, 2021, https://www.cancer.gov/about-cancer/treatment/clinical-trials/search/v?id=NCI-2020-01067&r=1.

13. You can review a current summary of studies at "Cannabis and Cannabinoids (PDQ®)–Health Professional Version," National Institutes of Health, National Cancer Institute, Cancer.gov, updated June 3, 2021, https://www.cancer.gov/about-cancer/treatment/cam/hp/cannabis-pdq.

14. Per "Gwyneth Paltrow: Charity Work, Events and Causes," *Look to the Stars*, accessed June 17, 2020, https://www.looktothestars.org/celebrity/gwyneth-paltrow.

15. And what the *hell* is up with this obsession with vaginas??

16. Amy B. Wang, "Gwyneth Paltrow's Goop Touted the 'Benefits' of Putting a Jade Egg in Your Vagina. Now It Must Pay," *Washington Post*, September 5, 2018, https://www.washingtonpost.com/health/2018/09/05/gwyneth-paltrows-goop-touted-benefits-putting-jade-egg-your-vagina-now-it-must-pay/.

17. Jen Gunter, "Dear Gwyneth Paltrow, I'm a GYN and Your Vaginal Jade Eggs Are a Bad Idea," *Dr. Jen Gunter*, January 17, 2017, https://drjengunter.com/2017/01/17/dear-gwyneth-paltrow-im-a-gyn-and-your-vaginal-jade-eggs-are-a-bad-idea/. And also check out Jen Gunter, *The Vagina Bible: The Vulva and the Vagina; Separating the Myth from the Medicine* (New York: Citadel Press, 2019).

18. Anna Merlan, "The 'Energy Worker' Seen on Goop Has Implied that His Treatments Can Disappear Breast Cancer," Life, *Vice*, January 28, 2020, https://www.vice.com/en/article/939kk8/the-energy-worker-seen-on-goop-has -implied-that-his-treatments-can-disappear-breast-cancer.

19. Merlan, "The 'Energy Worker' Seen on Goop."

20. S. M. Kramer, "Fact or Fiction? Underwire Bras Cause Cancer," The Sciences, *Scientific American*, April 19, 2007, https://www.scientificamerican .com/article/fact-or-fiction-underwire-bras-cause-cancer/.

21. Victoria Forster, "Gwyneth Paltrow's Goop Should Stay in Its Lane, Far Away from People with Cancer," *Forbes*, January 7, 2020, https://www.forbes .com/sites/victoriaforster/2020/01/07/gwyneth-paltrows-goop-should-stay-in -its-lane-far-away-from-people-with-cancer/.

22. Forster, "Gwyneth Paltrow's Goop." And visit Forster's website at http://www.drvickyforster.com/.

23. Check it out at https://feastingonveggies.wordpress.com/.

24. Yvette d'Entremont, "David Avocado Wolfe Is the Biggest Asshole in the Multiverse," *The Outline*, August 7, 2017, https://theoutline.com/ post/1951/david-avocado-wolfe-is-the-biggest-asshole-in-the-multiverse. And check out her other writing at https://scibabe.com/.

25. See "'Chemtrails' Not Real, Say Leading Atmospheric Science Experts," Carnegie Science, August 12, 2016, https://carnegiescience.edu/node/2077.

26. Dan Broadbent, "The David Avocado Wolfe Effect," A *Science Enthusiast*, June 20, 2015, https://ascienceenthusiast.com/the-david-avocado-wolfe -effect/.

27. I am loath to link to his site, but in the interest of providing proof, see David Wolfe, "Vitamin B17 May Treat Cancer, but Is Illegal in the US!" DavidWolfe.com, accessed June 17, 2021, https://www.davidwolfe.com/ vitamin-b17-kills-cancer-illegal-us/.

28. "Laetrile (Amygdalin or Vitamin B17)," Cancer Research UK, last reviewed October 17, 2018, https://www.cancerresearchuk.org/about-cancer/ cancer-in-general/treatment/complementary-alternative-therapies/individual -therapies/laetrile.

29. David Wolfe, "Medicinal Mushroom Benefits: What Does the Science Have to Say?" DavidWolfe.com, June 3, 2019, https://shop.davidwolfe.com/ blogs/health/medicinal-mushrooms.

30. Satoru Arata et al., "Continuous Intake of the Chaga Mushroom (*Inonotus obliquus*) Aqueous Extract Suppresses Cancer Progression and Maintains Body Temperature in Mice," *Heliyon* 2, no. 5 (May 2016): e00111, https://doi.org/10.1016/j.heliyon.2016.e00111, https://www.ncbi.nlm.nih.gov/ pubmed/27441282.

31. Arata et al., "Continuous Intake of the Chaga Mushroom."

32. Wolfe, "Medicinal Mushroom Benefits."

33. Ananya Mandal, "Darla Shine Joins Anti-vaccination Campaigners, Increases Threat of Measles Outbreak in the US," News Medical, February 15, 2019, https://www.news-medical.net/news/20190215/Darla-Shine-joins-anti-vaccination-campaigners-increases-threat-of-measles-outbreak-in-US.aspx.

34. "The Iron Lung and Other Equipment," Whatever Happened to Polio? Smithsonian National Museum of American History, accessed June 17, 2021, https://amhistory.si.edu/polio/howpolio/ironlung.htm.

35. "Polio Elimination in the United States," Centers for Disease Control, CDC.gov, last reviewed October 25, 2019, https://www.cdc.gov/polio/what-is-polio/polio-us.html.

36. Mandal, "Darla Shine Joins Anti-vaccination Campaigners."

37. "Correlation and Causation: Lesson," Khan Academy, accessed June 17, 2021, https://www.khanacademy.org/test-prep/praxis-math/praxis-math-lessons/gtp--praxis-math--lessons--statistics-and-probability/a/gtp--praxis-math--article--correlation-and-causation—lesson, emphasis original.

38. Robyn M. Lucas and Rachael M. Rodney Harris, "On the Nature of Evidence and 'Proving' Causality: Smoking and Lung Cancer vs. Sun Exposure, Vitamin D and Multiple Sclerosis," International Journal of Environmental Research and Public Health 15, no. 8 (August 12, 2018): 1726, https://doi.org/10.3390/ijerph15081726, https://www.ncbi.nlm.nih.gov/pubmed/30103527.

39. Stephen J. Russell et al., "Oncolytic Measles Virotherapy and Opposition to Measles Vaccination," Mayo Clinic Procedings 94, no. 9 (2019): 1834–39, https://doi.org/https://doi.org/10.1016/j.mayocp.2019.05.006, https://www.mayoclinicproceedings.org/article/S0025-6196(19)30462-8/pdf.

40. Russell et al., "Oncolytic Measles Virotherapy."

41. The PubMed database is available online at https://pubmed.ncbi.nlm.nih.gov/.

42. Check out the American Cancer Society's full list of red flags at "The Truth about Alternative Medical Treatments," Cancer.org, January 30, 2019, https://www.cancer.org/latest-news/the-truth-about-alternative-medical-treatments.html.

Chapter Eleven

1. You can find it at Dana M. Brantley-Sieders, "(Sensational) Headlines: How to Interpret Science News," Talking Tatas, January 23, 2020, https://talkingtatas.com/2020/01/23/beyond-the-sensational-headlines-how-to-interpret-science-news/.

2. Read the whole paper at Wenqiang Song et al., "Targeting EphA2 Impairs Cell Cycle Progression and Growth of Basal-like/Triple-Negative Breast Cancers," *Oncogene* 36, no. 40 (October 5, 2017): 5620–30, https://doi .org/10.1038/onc.2017.170, https://www.ncbi.nlm.nih.gov/pubmed/28581527.

3. Read more about "Patient-Derived Xenographs: PDX Models" at Charles River Laboratories, CRiver.com, accessed June 17, 2021, https://www.criver .com/products-services/discovery-services/pharmacology-studies/oncology -immuno-oncology-studies/oncology-study-models/patient-derived-xenografts -pdx-models.

4. Access PubMed Central's online portal at https://www.ncbi.nlm.nih.gov/ pmc/about/intro/.

5. Find out more about them at "Programs: Bicycle Conjugates," Bicycle Therapeutics, accessed June 17, 2021, https://www.bicycletherapeutics.com/ programs/#bicycle-conjugates.

6. Find out more about the clinical trial at "Study BT5528-100 in Patients with Advanced Solid Tumors Associated with EphA2 Expression," US National Library of Medicine, ClinicalTrials.gov, National Institutes of Health, accessed June 24, 2021, https://clinicaltrials.gov/ct2/show/NCT04180371.

7. Better cited as Iftiin Hassan Mohamed et al., "Polyphenol Rich Botanicals Used as Food Supplements Interfere with EphA2-ephrinA1 System," *Pharmacological Research* 64, no. 5 (November 2011): 464–70, https://doi.org/10.1016/j .phrs.2011.06.008, https://www.ncbi.nlm.nih.gov/pubmed/21742039.

8. Evan Andrews, "7 Unusual Ancient Medical Techniques," History Stories, History.com, accessed June 17, 2021, https://www.history.com/news/ 7-unusual-ancient-medical-techniques.

9. They're online at https://pubpeer.com/.

Chapter Twelve

1. Though some of the speakers might be hungover too.

2. Check out her memoir, *Becoming* (New York: Crown, 2018).

3. Rita Colwell and Sharon Bertsch McGrayne, *A Lab of One's Own: One Woman's Personal Journey through Sexism in Science* (New York: Simon and Schuster, 2020).

4. Rita Colwell, "Women Scientists Have the Evidence about Sexism," *The Atlantic*, August 30, 2020, https://www.theatlantic.com/ideas/archive/2020/08/ women-scientists-have-evidence-about-sexism-science/615823/.

5. Which she shouldn't need, but women aren't given the benefit of the doubt. Look how long it took Bill Cosby's many accusers to be taken seriously.

Chapter Thirteen

1. American Cancer Society, *Breast Cancer Facts and Figures, 2019–2020,* 10.

2. The above direct quotations are from, in order, page 33 of Suzanne H. Reuben, Erin L. Milliken, and Lisa J. Paradis, *The Future of Cancer Research: Accelerating Scientific Innovation,* President's Cancer Panel Annual Report, 2010–2011 ([Bethesda, MD]: US Department of Health and Human Services and the National Institutes of Health, 2012), https://deainfo.nci.nih.gov/advisory/pcp/annualreports/pcp10-11rpt/FullReport.pdf; page 4 of "Program Announcement for the Department of Defense, Defense Health Program, Congressionally Directed Medical Research Programs, Breast Cancer Research Program Breakthrough Award Levels 1 and 2," US Department of Defense, CDMRP, accessed June 17, 2021, https://cdmrp.army.mil/funding/pa/fy19-bcrp-bta12.pdf; and the mission statement from the Center for Strategic Scientific Initiatives' Provocative Questions Initiative, at "Provocative Questions," National Institutes of Health, National Cancer Institute, Cancer.gov, accessed June 17, 2021, https://provocativequestions.nci.nih.gov/about-pqs/mission.

3. For more on the seven known viruses that cause human cancer, see Kellie Bramlet Blackburn, "7 Viruses that Cause Cancer," MD Anderson Cancer Center, August 2018, https://www.mdanderson.org/publications/focused-on-health/7-viruses-that-cause-cancer.h17-1592202.html.

4. See Sue McGreevey, "Why Antiangiogenesis Fails: Team Finds Possible Mechanism behind Resistance to Cancer Treatment," News and Research, Harvard Medical School, October 12, 2016, https://hms.harvard.edu/news/why-antiangiogenesis-fails.

5. Belinda Seto, "Rapamycin and mTOR: A Serendipitous Discovery and Implications for Breast Cancer," *Clinical and Translational Medicine* 1, no. 1 (November 15, 2012): e29, https://doi.org/10.1186/2001-1326-1-29, https://www.ncbi.nlm.nih.gov/pubmed/23369283.

6. David B. Vaught et al., "EphA2 Is a Clinically Relevant Target for Breast Cancer Bone Metastatic Disease," *JBMR Plus* 5, no. 4 (March 9, 2021): e10465, doi: 10.1002/jbm4.10465, https://pubmed.ncbi.nlm.nih.gov/33869989/.

7. Norman E. Sharpless, "Funding from Congress Allows NCI to Raise Grants Payline," National Institutes of Health, National Cancer Institute, Cancer.gov, February 4, 2021, https://www.cancer.gov/grants-training/nci-bottom-line-blog/2021/funding-from-congress-allows-nci-to-raise-grants-payline.

Chapter Fourteen

1. "About Chronic Diseases," Centers for Disease Control and Prevention, CDC.gov, last reviewed April 28, 2021, https://www.cdc.gov/chronicdisease/about/index.htm.
2. Check her out at https://thebloggess.com/.
3. Jenny Lawson, *Let's Pretend This Never Happened: A Mostly True Memoir* (New York: Putnam Adult, 2012).
4. Jenny Lawson talks about this candidly in her second memoir, *Furiously Happy: A Funny Book about Horrible Things* (New York: Flatiron Books, 2017).
5. "Chronic Illness," Health Library, Cleveland Clinic (website), May 10, 2021, https://my.clevelandclinic.org/health/articles/4062-chronic-illness.
6. Rebecca Joy Stanborough, "What Are Cognitive Distortions and How Can You Change These Thinking Patterns? 'Should' Statements," *Healthline*, December 18, 2019, https://www.healthline.com/health/cognitive-distortions#should-statements.
7. The Women's Institute for Sexual Health is online at https://www.wishnashville.com/.
8. Learn more at "Revaree," Bonafide (website), accessed June 17, 2021, https://hellobonafide.com/products/revaree.
9. Learn more at "Ristela," Bonafide (website), accessed June 25, 2021, https://hellobonafide.com/products/ristela.
10. Learn more at "Vaginal Atrophy," Health Library, Cleveland Clinic, last reviewed October 27, 2020, https://my.clevelandclinic.org/health/diseases/15500-vaginal-atrophy.
11. Heather Currie, "Urogenital Problems," in collaboration with the medical advisory council of the British Menopause Society, Women's Health Concern (website), last reviewed August 2020, https://www.womens-health-concern.org/help-and-advice/factsheets/urogenital-problems/.
12. "Find Your Representative" at https://www.house.gov/representatives/find-your-representative.
13. Visit the American Association of Sexuality Educators, Counselors and Therapists online at https://www.aasect.org/.

Chapter Fifteen

1. For example, "Twelve Things to Never Say to Someone Who Has Cancer," chat thread, Cancer Research UK, accessed June 17, 2021, https://www.cancerresearchuk.org/about-cancer/cancer-chat/thread/12-things-never-to-say-to-someone-who-has-cancer (log-in required); and Sarah Crow, "20

Things You Should Never Say to Someone Battling Cancer," BestLifeOnline. com, September 13, 2018, https://bestlifeonline.com/cancer-support/.

2. Sean L. McCarthy, "Jon Stewart Offers Rally to Restore Sanity Tips: Among Them, You Can Watch on Comedy Central or Online," *The Comic's Comic*, October 13, 2010, https://thecomicscomic.com/2010/10/13/jon-stew art-offers-rally-to-restore-sanity-tips-among-them-you-can-watch-on-comedy -central-or-online/.

3. Zuckerman quoted in Elizabeth Yuko, "How to Avoid Toxic Positivity (And Handle It When It Comes Your Way)," *Lifehacker*, September 6, 2020, https://lifehacker.com/how-to-avoid-toxic-positivity-and-handle-it-when-it -co-1844966691.

4. Yuko, "How to Avoid Toxic Positivity."

Chapter Sixteen

1. "Distant Recurrence Risk of Hormone-Receptor-Positive Breast Cancer Steady 20 Years After Initial Diagnosis," Breastcancer.org, November 13, 2017, https://www.breastcancer.org/research-news/distant-recurrence-risk -steady-20-years-later.

2. Paula Dobosz and Tomasz Dzieciątkowski, "The Intriguing History of Cancer Immunotherapy," *Frontiers in Immunology* 10 (December 17, 2019): 2965, https://doi.org/10.3389/fimmu.2019.02965, https://www.ncbi .nlm.nih.gov/pubmed/31921205, https://www.frontiersin.org/articles/10.3389/ fimmu.2019.02965/full.

3. Heidi Ledford, Holly Else, and Matthew Warren, "Cancer Immunologists Scoop Medicine Nobel Prize," *Nature*, October 1, 2018, https://www.nature. com/articles/d41586-018-06751-0.

4. See American Cancer Society medical and editorial content team, "Immunotherapy for Breast Cancer," Treating Breast Cancer, American Cancer Society, Cancer.org, last revised December 3, 2020, https://www.cancer.org/ cancer/breast-cancer/treatment/immunotherapy.html.

5. Behzad Rowshanravan, Neil Halliday, and David M. Sansom, "CTLA-4: A Moving Target in Immunotherapy," *Blood* 131, no. 1 (January 4, 2018): 58–67, https://doi.org/10.1182/blood-2017-06-741033, https://www.ncbi.nlm .nih.gov/pubmed/29118008.

6. Devon Carter, "Does Immunotherapy Treat Breast Cancer?" MD Anderson Center (website), University of Texas, March 26, 2021, https://www .mdanderson.org/cancerwise/does-immunotherapy-treat-breast-cancer.h00 -159385101.html.

7. Cheng Zhang et al., "Engineering CAR-T Cells," *Biomarker Research* 5 (June 24, 2017): 22, https://doi.org/10.1186/s40364-017-0102-y, https://www.ncbi.nlm.nih.gov/pubmed/28652918.

8. Yonggui Tian et al., "Gene Modification Strategies for Next-Generation CAR T Cells against Solid Cancers," *Journal of Hematology and Oncology* 13, no. 1 (May 18, 2020): 54, https://doi.org/10.1186/s13045-020-00890-6, https://pubmed.ncbi.nlm.nih.gov/32423475/.

9. See "Vaccine Types," Office of Infectious Diseases and HIV/AIDS Policy, HHS.gov, Vaccines.gov, April 29, 2021, https://www.vaccines.gov/basics/types.

10. For more information on the COVID vaccines, see my blog post, Dana M. Brantley-Sieders, "Getting to Know the COVID-19 Vaccines!" *Talking Tatas*, January 13, 2021, https://talkingtatas.com/2021/01/13/getting-to-know-the-covid-19-vaccines/.

11. NCI staff, "Large Study Confirms that HPV Vaccine Prevents Cervical Cancer," National Institutes of Health, National Cancer Institute, Cancer.gov, October 14, 2020, https://www.cancer.gov/news-events/cancer-currents-blog/2020/hpv-vaccine-prevents-cervical-cancer-sweden-study.

12. Caroline Tein, "FDA Clears Breast Cancer Vaccine for Clinical Trials," Health News, *Verywell Health*, January 8, 2021, https://www.verywellhealth.com/breast-cancer-vaccine-greenlit-clinical-trials-5094403.

13. NCI staff, "Large Study Confirms that HPV Vaccine Prevents Cervical Cancer," National Institutes of Health, National Cancer Institute, Cancer.gov, October 14, 2020, https://www.cancer.gov/news-events/cancer-currents-blog/2020/hpv-vaccine-prevents-cervical-cancer-sweden-study.

14. Caroline Tein, "FDA Clears Breast Cancer Vaccine for Clinical Trials," Health News, *Verywell Health*, January 8, 2021, https://www.verywellhealth.com/breast-cancer-vaccine-greenlit-clinical-trials-5094403.

15. Julia Evangelou Strait, "Breast Cancer Vaccine Shows Promise in Small Clinical Trial," Siteman Cancer Center, Washington University School of Medicine, accessed June 17, 2021, https://siteman.wustl.edu/breast-cancer-vaccine-shows-promise-in-small-clinical-trial/.

16. "Measles Virus-Based Immunovirotherapy in the Treatment of Metastatic Breast Cancer," Mayo Clinic Breast Cancer Spore, Mayo.edu, accessed June 17, 2021, https://www.mayo.edu/research/centers-programs/cancer-research/research-programs/womens-cancer-program/breast-cancer-spore/research-projects/measles-virus-based-immunovirotherapy-treatment-metastatic-breast-cancer.

Bibliography

Adams, Mike. "Science Tells Us Marijuana Doesn't Kill Cancer, So Does Real Life." *Forbes*, October 8, 2018. https://www.forbes.com/sites/mikeadams/2018/10/08/science-tells-us-marijuana-doesnt-kill-cancer-so-does-real-life.

AMBOSS. "Cell Cycle and Cancer: Phases, Hallmarks, and Development." Video. YouTube, uploaded April 27, 2018. https://www.youtube.com/watch?v=e0lNk-2Il_M.

American Association for Cancer Research. *AACR Cancer Disparities Progress Report 2020: Achieving the Bold Vision of Health Equity for Racial and Ethnic Minorities and Other Underserved Populations.* Philadelphia: American Association for Cancer Research, 2020. http://www.CancerDisparitiesProgressReport.org/ and https://cancerprogressreport.aacr.org/wp-content/uploads/sites/2/2020/09/AACR_CDPR_2020.pdf.

———. "Advances in Modeling Cancer in Mice: Technology, Biology, and Beyond." Video. First presented at the AACR Conference on Advances on Modeling Cancer in Mice: Technology, Biology, and Beyond, Orlando, FL, September 24–27, 2017. https://www.aacr.org/blog/2017/09/21/how-mouse-models-pave-the-way-to-precision-cancer-medicine/

American Association for Cancer Research press office. "How Mouse Models Pave the Way to Precision Cancer Medicine." AACR.org blog, September 21, 2019. https://www.aacr.org/blog/2017/09/21/how-mouse-models-pave-the-way-to-precision-cancer-medicine/.

American Breast Cancer Foundation. "Breast Cancer Assistance Program." Accessed June 25, 2021. https://www.abcf.org/programs/breast-cancer-assistance-program.

American Cancer Society. *Breast Cancer Facts and Figures, 2019–2020.* Atlanta: American Cancer Society, Inc., 2019. https://www.cancer.org/content/dam/cancer-org/research/cancer-facts-and-statistics/breast-cancer-facts-and-figures/breast-cancer-facts-and-figures-2019-2020.pdf.

———. "Breast Reconstruction Surgery." Cancer.org, accessed June 25, 2021. https://www.cancer.org/cancer/breast-cancer/reconstruction-surgery.html.

———. *Cancer Facts and Figures, 2020.* Atlanta: American Cancer Society, 2020. https://www.cancer.org/content/dam/cancer-org/research/cancer-facts-and-statistics/annual-cancer-facts-and-figures/2020/cancer-facts-and-figures-2020.pdf.

———. "Estimates for 2021." Cancer Statistics Center, Cancer.org, accessed July 15, 2021. https://cancerstatisticscenter.cancer.org/?_ga=2.27173118.2100259821.1626382499-2110999834.1626382499#!/.

American Cancer Society medical and editorial content team. "Breast Cancer HER2 Status," American Cancer Society, Cancer.org, last revised September 20, 2019. https://www.cancer.org/cancer/breast-cancer/understanding-a-breast-cancer-diagnosis/breast-cancer-her2-status.html.

———. "Breast MRI." American Cancer Society, Cancer.org, last revised October 3, 2019. https://www.cancer.org/cancer/breast-cancer/screening-tests-and-early-detection/breast-mri-scans.html.

———. "Chemo Brain." American Cancer Society, Cancer.org, last revised February 1, 2020. https://www.cancer.org/treatment/treatments-and-side-effects/physical-side-effects/changes-in-mood-or-thinking/chemo-brain.html.

———. "Hormone Therapy for Breast Cancer." American Cancer Society, Cancer.org, last revised September 18, 2019. https://www.cancer.org/cancer/breast-cancer/treatment/hormone-therapy-for-breast-cancer.html.

———. "Immunotherapy for Breast Cancer." Treating Breast Cancer. American Cancer Society, Cancer.org, last revised December 3, 2020. https://www.cancer.org/cancer/breast-cancer/treatment/immunotherapy.html.

———. "Radiation for Breast Cancer." American Cancer Society, Cancer.org, last revised September 19, 2019. https://www.cancer.org/cancer/breast-cancer/treatment/radiation-for-breast-cancer.html.

———. "Take a Moment with Meditation." American Cancer Society, Cancer.org, June 2, 2020. https://www.cancer.org/latest-news/take-a-moment-with-meditation.html.

———. "Triple-Negative Breast Cancer." American Cancer Society, Cancer.org, last revised January 27, 2021. https://www.cancer.org/cancer/breast

-cancer/understanding-a-breast-cancer-diagnosis/types-of-breast-cancer/
triple-negative.html.

———. "The Truth about Alternative Medical Treatments." Cancer.org, January 30, 2019. https://www.cancer.org/latest-news/the-truth-about-alterna
tive-medical-treatments.html.

American Medical Association. "Reducing Disparities in Health Care." Patient Support and Advocacy. Accessed June 17, 2021. https://www.ama-assn.org/
delivering-care/patient-support-advocacy/reducing-disparities-health-care.

American Psychological Association. "What Is Cognitive Behavioral Therapy?" APA.org, July 2017. https://www.apa.org/ptsd-guideline/patients-and
-families/cognitive-behavioral.

American Society of Breast Surgeons. "Fibroadenoma." Breast360.org, accessed June 17, 2021. https://breast360.org/topic/2015/10/24/fibroadenoma/.

Andrews, Evan. "7 Unusual Ancient Medical Techniques." History Stories. History.com, accessed June 17, 2021. https://www.history.com/news/7
-unusual-ancient-medical-techniques.

Anstett, Patricia. *Breast Cancer Surgery and Reconstruction: What's Right for You.* Photography by Kathleen Galligan. Lanham, MD: Rowman & Littlefield, 2016.

Arata, Satoru, Jun Watanabe, Masako Maeda, Masato Yamamoto, Hideto Matsuhashi, Mamiko Mochizuki, Nobuyuki Kagami, Kazuho Honda, and Masahiro Inagaki. "Continuous Intake of the Chaga Mushroom (*Inonotus obliquus*) Aqueous Extract Suppresses Cancer Progression and Maintains Body Temperature in Mice." *Heliyon* 2, no. 5 (May 2016): e00111. https://
doi.org/10.1016/j.heliyon.2016.e00111. https://www.ncbi.nlm.nih.gov/
pubmed/27441282.

Aspan, Maria. "'We Can't Ever Go to the Doctor without Our Guard Down': Why Black Women Are 40% More Likely to Die of Breast Cancer." *Fortune*, June 30, 2020. https://fortune.com/2020/06/30/black-women-breast-cancer
-mortality-racism-healthcare-pandemic/.

AstraZeneca. "DMC Has Concluded that OlympiA Trial of Lynparza Crossed Superiority Boundary for Invasive Disease-Free Survival vs. Placebo at Planned Interim Analysis." News release. February 17, 2021. https://
www.astrazeneca.com/media-centre/press-releases/2021/olympia-trial-of
-lynparza-idmc-recommend-early-analysis.html.

Bazell, Robert. *Her-2: The Making of Herceptin, a Revolutionary Treatment for Breast Cancer.* Edited by Ann Godoff. New York: Random House, 2011.

Berg, Wendie A., Jeremy M. Berg, Edward A. Sickles, Elizabeth S. Burnside, Margarita L. Zuley, Robert D. Rosenberg, and Cindy S. Lee. "Cancer Yield and Patterns of Follow-Up for BI-RADS Category 3 after Screening Mammography Recall in the National Mammography Database." *Radiology* 296, no. 1 (July 2020): 32–41. https://doi.org/10.1148/radiol.2020192641 . https://www.ncbi.nlm.nih.gov/pubmed/32427557.

Bernhardt, Sarah M., Pallave Dasari, David Walsh, Amanda R. Townsend, Timothy J. Price, and Wendy V. Ingman. "Hormonal Modulation of Breast Cancer Gene Expression: Implications for Intrinsic Subtyping in Premenopausal Women." *Frontiers in Oncology* 6 (November 2016): 241. https://doi.org/10.3389/fonc.2016.00241. https://www.ncbi.nlm.nih.gov/ pubmed/27896218.

Bicycle Therapeutics. "Programs: Bicycle Conjugates." Accessed June 17, 2021. https://www.bicycletherapeutics.com/programs/#bicycle-conjugates.

Bidot, Samuel, and Xiaoxian (Bill) Li. "Breast: Other Benign Tumors; Intraductal Papilloma." PathologyOutlines.com, Inc., last updated June 25, 2021. https://www.pathologyoutlines.com/topic/breastpapilloma.html.

Blackburn, Kellie Bramlet. "7 Viruses that Cause Cancer." MD Anderson Cancer Center, August 2018. https://www.mdanderson.org/publications/ focused-on-health/7-viruses-that-cause-cancer.h17-1592202.html.

Blakemore, Erin. "1,800 Studies Later, Scientists Conclude Homeopathy Doesn't Work." Smart News. *Smithsonian Magazine*, March 11, 2015. https://www.smithsonianmag.com/smart-news/1800-studies-later-scientists-conclude-homeopathy-doesnt-work-180954534/.

Boehmer, Ulrike. "LGBT Populations' Barriers to Cancer Care." *Seminars in Oncology Nursing* 34, no. 1 (February 2018): 21–29. https://doi.org/10.1016/j .soncn.2017.11.002. https://www.ncbi.nlm.nih.gov/pubmed/29338894.

Bonafide. "Revaree." Accessed June 17, 2021. https://hellobonafide.com/ products/revaree.

———. "Ristela." Accessed June 25, 2021. https://hellobonafide.com/products/ ristela.

Brady, Donita C., and Ashanti T. Weeraratna. "The Race toward Equity: Increasing Racial Diversity in Cancer Research and Cancer Care." *Cancer Discovery* 10, no. 10 (Oct 2020): 1451–54. https://doi.org/10.1158/2159 -8290.CD-20-1193. https://www.ncbi.nlm.nih.gov/pubmed/32816861.

Brantley, Dana M., Fiona E. Yull, Rebecca S. Muraoka, Donna J. Hicks, Christopher M. Cook, and Lawrence D. Kerr. "Dynamic Expression and Activity of NF-kappaB during Post-natal Mammary Gland Morphogenesis." *Mechanisms of Development* 97, nos. 1–2 (October 2000): 149–55. https:// doi.org/10.1016/S0925-4773(00)00405-6.

Brantley-Sieders, Dana M. "Getting to Know the COVID-19 Vaccines!" *Talking Tatas*, January 13, 2021. https://talkingtatas.com/2021/01/13/getting-to -know-the-covid-19-vaccines/.

———. "Lumpectomy versus Mastectomy: I've Had 'Em Both and I'm Telling You All about It." *Talking Tatas*, August 9, 2020. https://talkingtatas .com/2020/08/09/lumpectomy-versus-mastectomy-ive-had-em-both-and -im-telling-you-all-about-it/.

———. "Science Break! Outreach: Getting High School Students Excited about Cancer Research." *Talking Tatas*, January 20, 2020. https://talkingta tas.com/2020/01/20/science-break-outreach-getting-high-school-students -excited-about-cancer-research/.

———. "(Sensational) Headlines: How to Interpret Science News." *Talking Tatas*, January 23, 2020. https://talkingtatas.com/2020/01/23/beyond-the -sensational-headlines-how-to-interpret-science-news/.

Brantley-Sieders, Dana M., Kang-Hsien Fan, Sandra L. Deming-Halverson, Yu Shyr, and Rebecca S. Cook. "Local Breast Cancer Spatial Patterning: A Tool for Community Health Resource Allocation to Address Local Disparities in Breast Cancer Mortality." *PLoS One* 7, no. 9 (September 2012): e45238. https://doi.org/10.1371/journal.pone.0045238. https://www.ncbi .nlm.nih.gov/pubmed/23028869.

Breast Cancer Now. "Caring for Scars after Breast Cancer Surgery." News and Personal Stories. March 8, 2017. https://breastcancernow.org/about-us/ news-personal-stories/caring-scars-after-breast-cancer-surgery.

———. "Intraductal Papilloma." Last reviewed December 2018. https:// breastcancernow.org/information-support/have-i-got-breast-cancer/benign -breast-conditions/intraductal-papilloma.

Breastcancer.org. "Breast Reconstruction." Last modified May 15, 2021. https://www.breastcancer.org/treatment/surgery/reconstruction.

———. "Breast Self-Exam." Last modified October 24, 2019. https://www .breastcancer.org/symptoms/testing/types/self_exam.

———. "Distant Recurrence Risk of Hormone-Receptor-Positive Breast Cancer Steady 20 Years After Initial Diagnosis." November 13, 2017. https://www.breastcancer.org/research-news/distant-recurrence-risk-steady -20-years-later.

———. "Fertility Issues." Last modified July 22, 2020. https://www.breastcan cer.org/treatment/side_effects/fertility_issues.

———. "HER2 Status." Breastcancer.org, last modified September 21, 2020. https://www.breastcancer.org/symptoms/diagnosis/her2.

———. "Hormone Receptor Status." Last modified September 21, 2020. https://www.breastcancer.org/symptoms/diagnosis/hormone_status.

———. "How Does Complementary Medicine Work?" Last modified May 5, 2020. https://www.breastcancer.org/treatment/comp_med/what_is_it/ how_it_works.

———. "How Is Chemotherapy Given?" Last modified March 25, 2020. https://www.breastcancer.org/treatment/chemotherapy/process/how.

———. "How to Read Hormone Receptor Test Results." Last modified September 21, 2020. https://www.breastcancer.org/symptoms/diagnosis/hormone_status/read_results.

———. "Lumpectomy." Last modified March 9, 2019. https://www.breastcancer.org/treatment/surgery/lumpectomy.

———. "Many Women Treated with Brachytherapy Aren't Good Candidates." Research News. December 19, 2011. https://www.breastcancer.org/research-news/20111219.

———. "Meditation." Last modified May 5, 2020. https://www.breastcancer.org/treatment/comp_med/types/meditation.

———. "Support Groups." Last modified May 5, 2020. https://www.breastcancer.org/treatment/comp_med/types/group.

———. "Triple-Negative Breast Cancer." Last modified April 9, 2021. https://www.breastcancer.org/symptoms/diagnosis/trip_neg.

———. "Using HRT (Hormone Replacement Therapy)." Last modified April 21, 2021. https://www.breastcancer.org/risk/factors/hrt.

———. "What Is Mastectomy?" Last modified October 29, 2020. https://www.breastcancer.org/treatment/surgery/mastectomy/what_is.

Broadbent, Dan. "The David Avocado Wolfe Effect." *A Science Enthusiast*, June 20, 2015. https://ascienceenthusiast.com/the-david-avocado-wolfe-effect/.

Brown, DeNeen L. "'You've Got Bad Blood': The Horror of the Tuskegee Syphilis Experiment." Retropolis. *Washington Post*, May 16, 2017. https://www.washingtonpost.com/news/retropolis/wp/2017/05/16/youve-got-bad-blood-the-horror-of-the-tuskegee-syphilis-experiment/.

Campbell, Jean. "Surgical Drains after Breast Surgery." Verywell Health, March 23, 2021. https://www.verywellhealth.com/managing-your-surgical-drains-following-breast-surgery-4021630.

Campbell, Kirsteen J., and Stephen W. G. Tait. "Targeting BCL-2 Regulated Apoptosis in Cancer." *Open Biology* 8, no. 5 (May 2018): 180002. https://doi.org/10.1098/rsob.180002. https://www.ncbi.nlm.nih.gov/pubmed/29769323.

Cancer Health staff. "Finding Inspiration in Patton Oswalt's 'It's Chaos. Be Kind.'" *Cancer Health* blog, November 10, 2017. https://www.cancerhealth.com/blog/finding-inspiration-in-patton-oswalt-its-chaos-be-kind.

CancerQuest. "Animated Introduction to Cancer Biology (Full Documentary)." Video. Emory University, Winship Cancer Institute. Accessed June 18, 2021. http://www.cancerquest.org/patients/what-cancer.

Cancer Research UK. "Laetrile (Amygdalin or Vitamin B17)." Last reviewed October 17, 2018. https://www.cancerresearchuk.org/about-cancer/cancer -in-general/treatment/complementary-alternative-therapies/individual -therapies/laetrile.

———. "Twelve Things to Never Say to Someone Who Has Cancer." Chat thread. Accessed June 17, 2021. https://www.cancerresearchuk.org/about -cancer/cancer-chat/thread/12-things-never-to-say-to-someone-who-has -cancer (log-in required).

Cardiff, Robert D. "Validity of Mouse Mammary Tumour Models for Human Breast Cancer: Comparative Pathology." *Microscopy Research and Technique* 52, no. 2 (January 15 2001): 224–30. https://doi.org/10.1002/1097-0029(20010115)52:2<224::AID-JEMT1007>3.0.CO;2-A. https://www .ncbi.nlm.nih.gov/pubmed/11169869.

Cardiff, Robert D., and Sefton R. Wellings. "The Comparative Pathology of Human and Mouse Mammary Glands." *Journal of Mammary Gland Biology and Neoplasia* 4, no. 1 (January 1999): 105–22. https:// doi.org/10.1023/a:1018712905244. https://www.ncbi.nlm.nih.gov/ pubmed/10219910.

Cardiff, Robert D., Sonali Jindal, Piper M. Treuting, James J. Going, Barry Gusterson, and Henry J. Thompson. "Mammary Gland." In *Comparative Anatomy and Histology: A Mouse, Rat, and Human Atlas.* 2nd ed. Edited by Piper M. Treuting, Suzanne M. Dintzis, and Kathleen S. Montine, 487–510. London: Elsevier/Academic Press, 2018.

Carnegie Science. "'Chemtrails' Not Real, Say Leading Atmospheric Science Experts." August 12, 2016. https://carnegiescience.edu/node/2077.

Carter, Devon. "Does Immunotherapy Treat Breast Cancer?" MD Anderson Center (website), University of Texas, March 26, 2021. https://www .mdanderson.org/cancerwise/does-immunotherapy-treat-breast-cancer.h00 -159385101.html.

Center for Strategic Scientific Initiatives. "Provocative Questions." National Institutes of Health, National Cancer Institute, Cancer.gov, accessed June 17, 2021. https://provocativequestions.nci.nih.gov/about-pqs/mission.

Centers for Disease Control and Prevention. "About Chronic Diseases." CDC. gov, last reviewed April 28, 2021. https://www.cdc.gov/chronicdisease/ about/index.htm.

———. "Breast Cancer in Men." CDC.gov, last reviewed August 11, 2020. https://www.cdc.gov/cancer/breast/men/index.htm.

———. "Breast Cancer Screening Guidelines for Women." CDC.gov, last reviewed September 22, 2020. https://www.cdc.gov/cancer/breast/pdf/breast -cancer-screening-guidelines-508.pdf.

———. "Hereditary Breast Cancer and BRCA Genes." CDC.gov, last reviewed April 5, 2019. https://www.cdc.gov/cancer/breast/young_women/bringyour brave/hereditary_breast_cancer/.

———. "Polio Elimination in the United States." CDC.gov, last reviewed October 25, 2019. https://www.cdc.gov/polio/what-is-polio/polio-us.html

———. "What Are the Risk Factors for Breast Cancer?" CDC.gov, last reviewed September 14, 2020. https://www.cdc.gov/cancer/breast/basic_info/ risk_factors.htm.

Charles River Laboratories. "Patient-Derived Xenographs: PDX Models." CRiver.com, accessed June 17, 2021. https://www.criver.com/products-ser vices/discovery-services/pharmacology-studies/oncology-immuno-oncology -studies/oncology-study-models/patient-derived-xenografts-pdx-models.

Cheng, Chien-Jui, Yuh-Charn Lin, Ming-Tzu Tsai, Ching-Shyang Chen, Mao-Chih Hsieh, Chi-Long Chen, and Ruey-Bing Yang. "SCUBE2 Suppresses Breast Tumor Cell Poliferation and Confers a Favorable Prognosis in Invasive Breast Cancer." *Cancer Research* 69, no. 8 (April 15, 2009): 3634–41. https://doi.org/10.1158/0008-5472.CAN-08-3615. https://www .ncbi.nlm.nih.gov/pubmed/19369267.

Cianna Medical Group. "FDA Clears World's First and Only Wire-Free Radar Breast Tumor Localization System for Long Term Implant Capabilities." News release. November 13, 2017. https://www.ciannamedical.com/cianna_news _releases/fda-clears-worlds-first-wire-free-radar-breast-tumor-local ization-system-long-term-implant-capabilities/ (link inactive). Text available at https://www.globenewswire.com/en/news-release/2017/ 11/13/1185036/37185/en/FDA-Clears-World-s-First-and-Only-Wire-Free -Radar-Breast-Tumor-Localization-System-for-Long-Term-Implant-Capa bilities.html.

Cleveland Clinic. "Chronic Illness." Health Library. May 10, 2021. https:// my.clevelandclinic.org/health/articles/4062-chronic-illness.

———. "Vaginal Atrophy." Health Library. Last reviewed October 27, 2020. https://my.clevelandclinic.org/health/diseases/15500-vaginal-atrophy.

Colwell, Rita. "Women Scientists Have the Evidence about Sexism." *The Atlantic*, August 30, 2020. https://www.theatlantic.com/ideas/archive/2020/08/ women-scientists-have-evidence-about-sexism-science/615823/.

Colwell, Rita, and Sharon Bertsch McGrayne. *A Lab of One's Own: One Woman's Personal Journey through Sexism in Science.* New York: Simon and Schuster, 2020.

Crawley, Jacqueline N., Wolf-Dietrich Heyer, and Janine M. LaSalle. "Autism and Cancer Share Risk Genes, Pathways, and Drug Targets." *Trends in Genetics* 32, no. 3 (March 2016): 139–46. https://doi.org/10.1016/j .tig.2016.01.001. https://www.ncbi.nlm.nih.gov/pubmed/26830258.

Crow, Sarah. "20 Things You Should Never Say to Someone Battling Cancer." BestLifeOnline.com, September 13, 2018. https://bestlifeonline.com/cancer-support/.

Currie, Heather. "Urogenital Problems." Article written in collaboration with the medical advisory council of the British Menopause Society. Women's Health Concern (website), last reviewed August 2020. https://www.womens-health-concern.org/help-and-advice/factsheets/urogenital-problems/.

d'Entremont, Yvette. "David Avocado Wolfe Is the Biggest Asshole in the Multiverse." The Outline, August 7, 2017. https://theoutline.com/post/1951/david-avocado-wolfe-is-the-biggest-asshole-in-the-multiverse.

Darbro, Benjamin W., Rohini Singh, M. Bridget Zimmerman, Vinit B. Mahajan, and Alexander G. Bassuk. "Autism Linked to Increased Oncogene Mutations but Decreased Cancer Rate." PLoS One 11, no. 3 (March 2, 2016): e0149041. https://doi.org/10.1371/journal.pone.0149041. https://www.ncbi.nlm.nih.gov/pubmed/26934580.

Davenport, Liam. "Is There an Ideal Healthcare System for Treating Cancer?" Medscape Oncology, September 24, 2019. https://www.medscape.com/viewarticle/918795#vp_2.

de Blok, Christel J. M., Chantal M. Wiepjes, Nienke M. Nota, Klaartje van Engelen, Muriel A. Adank, Koen M. A. Dreijerink, Ellis Barbe, Inge R. H. M. Konings, and Martin den Heijer. "Breast Cancer Risk in Transgender People Receiving Hormone Treatment: Nationwide Cohort Study in the Netherlands." BMJ 365 (May 14, 2019): l1652. https://doi.org/10.1136/bmj.l1652. https://www.ncbi.nlm.nih.gov/pubmed/31088823.

Deering, Shelby. "Nature's 9 Most Powerful Medicinal Plants and the Science behind Them: Chamomile." Healthline, updated February 28, 2019. https://www.healthline.com/health/most-powerful-medicinal-plants#chamomile.

Dembosky, April. "Stop Blaming Tuskegee, Critics Say. It's Not an 'Excuse' for Current Medical Racism." NPR.org, March 23, 2021. https://www.npr.org/sections/health-shots/2021/03/23/974059870/stop-blaming-tuskegee-critics-say-its-not-an-excuse-for-current-medical-racism.

DePolo, Jamie. "Feminizing Hormones Linked to Higher Breast Cancer Risk in Trans Women, but Risk Still Lower than Average Woman's." Research News. Breastcancer.org, May 17, 2019. https://www.breastcancer.org/research-news/feminizing-hormones-increase-risk-in-trans-women.

Dobosz, Paula, and Tomasz Dzieciątkowski. "The Intriguing History of Cancer Immunotherapy." Frontiers in Immunology 10 (December 17, 2019): 2965. https://doi.org/10.3389/fimmu.2019.02965. https://www.ncbi.nlm.nih.gov/pubmed/31921205.

Forster, Victoria. "Gwyneth Paltrow's Goop Should Stay in Its Lane, Far Away from People with Cancer." *Forbes*, January 7, 2020. https://www.forbes.com/sites/victoriaforster/2020/01/07/gwyneth-paltrows-goop-should-stay-in-its-lane-far-away-from-people-with-cancer/.

Garg, Himani, Prerna Suri, Jagdish C. Gupta, G. P. Talwar, and Shweta Dubey. "Survivin: A Unique Target for Tumor Therapy." *Cancer Cell International* 16 (June 23, 2016): 49. https://doi.org/10.1186/s12935-016-0326-1. https://www.ncbi.nlm.nih.gov/pubmed/27340370.

Godlee, Fiona, Jane Smith, and Harvey Marcovitch. "Wakefield's Article Linking MMR Vaccine and Autism Was Fraudulent." *BMJ* 342 (January 5, 2011): c7452. https://doi.org/10.1136/bmj.c7452. https://www.ncbi.nlm.nih.gov/pubmed/21209060.

Goldberg, Sana. *How to Be a Patient: The Essential Guide to Navigating the World of Modern Medicine.* New York: HarperCollins, 2019.

Gunter, Jen. "Dear Gwyneth Paltrow, I'm a GYN and Your Vaginal Jade Eggs Are a Bad Idea." *Dr. Jen Gunter*, January 17, 2017. https://drjengunter.com/2017/01/17/dear-gwyneth-paltrow-im-a-gyn-and-your-vaginal-jade-eggs-are-a-bad-idea/.

———. *The Vagina Bible: The Vulva and the Vagina; Separating the Myth from the Medicine.* New York: Citadel Press, 2019.

Guthrie, Catherine. "These Cancer Patients Wanted to Get Rid of Their Breasts for Good. Their Doctors Had Other Ideas." *Cosmopolitan*, September 6, 2018. https://www.cosmopolitan.com/health-fitness/a22984204/breast-cancer-survivors-mastectomy-sexism/.

Hanahan, Douglas, and Robert A. Weinberg. "Hallmarks of Cancer: The Next Generation." *Cell* 144, no. 5 (March 4, 2011): 646–74. https://doi.org/10.1016/j.cell.2011.02.013. https://www.ncbi.nlm.nih.gov/pubmed/21376230.

Harris, Jay R., and Monica Morrow. "Breast-Conserving Therapy." In *Diseases of the Breast*, 5th ed., edited by Jay R. Harris, Marc E. Lippman, Monica Morrow, and C. Kent Osborne, 514–35. Philadelphia: Wolters Kluwer Health, 2014.

Herceptin.com. "Herceptin Dosing and Administration." Accessed March 15, 2021. https://www.herceptin.com/hcp/dosing-admin.html.

Hout, David R. "A Disease with Many Faces." Diagnostics. *The Pathologist*, May 3, 2019. https://thepathologist.com/diagnostics/a-disease-with-many-faces.

Hsu, Christine D., Xiaoyan Wang, David V. Habif Jr., Cynthia X. Ma, and Kimberly J. Johnson. "Breast Cancer Stage Variation and Survival in Association with Insurance Status and Sociodemographic Factors in US Women 18 to 64 Years Old." *Cancer* 123, no. 16 (August 15, 2017): 3125–31. https://doi.org/10.1002/cncr.30722. https://www.ncbi.nlm.nih .gov/pubmed/28440864.

Iezzoni, Lisa I., Sowmya R. Rao, Nicole D. Agaronnik, and Areej El-Jawahri. "Associations between Disability and Breast or Cervical Cancers, Accounting for Screening Disparities." *Medical Care* 59, no. 2 (February 1, 2021): 139–47. https://doi.org/10.1097/MLR.0000000000001449. https://www .ncbi.nlm.nih.gov/pubmed/33201087.

Jamison, Peter. "Anti-vaccination Leaders Sieze on Coronavirus to Push Resistance to Inoculation." Social Issues. *Washington Post*, May 5, 2020. https:// www.washingtonpost.com/dc-md-va/2020/05/05/anti-vaxxers-wakefield -coronavirus-vaccine/.

Jemal, Ahmedin, Anthony S. Robbins, Chun Chieh Lin, W. Dana Flanders, Carol E. DeSantis, Elizabeth M. Ward, and Rachel A. Freedman. "Factors that Contributed to Black-White Disparities in Survival among Nonelderly Women with Breast Cancer between 2004 and 2013." *Journal of Clinical Oncology* 36, no. 1 (January 1, 2018): 14–24. https://doi.org/10.1200/ JCO.2017.73.7932. https://www.ncbi.nlm.nih.gov/pubmed/29035645.

Jena, Manoj Kumar, and Jagadeesh Janjanam. "Role of Extracellular Matrix in Breast Cancer Development: A Brief Update." *F1000Research* 7 (March 5, 2018): 274. https://doi.org/10.12688/f1000research.14133.2. https://www .ncbi.nlm.nih.gov/pubmed/29983921.

Jenkins, Kristin. "Meta-Analysis: Recurrence Rates after Lumpectomy Have Improved." News. *Medscape*, May 4, 2018. https://www.medscape.com/ viewarticle/896185.

Johnson, Jon. "Depression after Surgery: What You Need to Know." *Medical News Today*, August 20, 2019. https://www.medicalnewstoday.com/ articles/317616.

Johnson, Skyler B., Henry S. Park, Cary P. Gross, and James B. Yu. "Complementary Medicine, Refusal of Conventional Cancer Therapy, and Survival among Patients with Curable Cancers." *JAMA Oncology* 4, no. 10 (October 1, 2018): 1375–81. https://doi.org/10.1001/jamaoncol.2018.2487. https:// www.ncbi.nlm.nih.gov/pubmed/30027204.

———. "Use of Alternative Medicine for Cancer and Its Impact on Survival." *Journal of the National Cancer Institute* 110, no. 1 (January 1, 2018). https://doi.org/10.1093/jnci/djx145. https://www.ncbi.nlm.nih.gov/ pubmed/28922780.

Khan Academy. "Correlation and Causation: Lesson." Accessed June 17, 2021. https://www.khanacademy.org/test-prep/praxis-math/praxis-math

-lessons/gtp--praxis-math--lessons--statistics-and-probability/a/gtp--praxis
-math--article--correlation-and-causation—lesson.

Kramer, S. M. "Fact or Fiction? Underwire Bras Cause Cancer." The Sciences. *Scientific American*, April 19, 2007. https://www.scientificamerican.com/article/fact-or-fiction-underwire-bras-cause-cancer/.

Kubala, Jillian. "7 Uses and Benefits of CBD Oil (Plus Side Effects)." *Healthline*, February 26, 2018. https://www.healthline.com/nutrition/cbd-oil-benefits.

Lawson, Jenny. *Furiously Happy: A Funny Book about Horrible Things*. New York: Flatiron Books, 2017.

———. *Let's Pretend This Never Happened: A Mostly True Memoir*. New York: Putnam Adult, 2012.

Ledford, Heidi, Holly Else, and Matthew Warren. "Cancer Immunologists Scoop Medicine Nobel Prize." *Nature*, October 1, 2018. https://www.nature.com/articles/d41586-018-06751-0.

Levy, Jane. "I've Just Been Diagnosed with Breast Cancer. Even with Insurance, I Have Many Out-of-Pocket Expenses. What Organizations Can Help Me?" Answer. Ask CancerCare Q&A, CancerCare.org, accessed June 25, 2021. https://www.cancercare.org/questions/136.

Lim, Elgee, Gerard Tarulli, Neil Portman, Theresa E. Hickey, Wayne D. Tilley, and Carlo Palmieri. "Pushing Estrogen Receptor Around in Breast Cancer." *Endocrine Related Cancer* 23, no. 12 (December 2016): T227–41. https://doi.org/10.1530/ERC-16-0427. https://www.ncbi.nlm.nih.gov/pubmed/27729416.

Living Beyond Breast Cancer. "Additional Resources." Get Support. Accessed June 25, 2021. https://www.lbbc.org/get-support/additional-resources.

Look to the Stars. "Gwyneth Paltrow: Charity Work, Events and Causes." Accessed June 17, 2020. https://www.looktothestars.org/celebrity/gwyneth-paltrow.

Losk, Katya, Rachel A. Freedman, Elizabeth A. Mittendorf, Zhenying Tan-Wasielewski, Lorenzo Trippa, and Tari A. King. "Oncotype DX Testing in Early-Stage Node-Positive Breast Cancer and Impact on Chemotherapy Use at a Comprehensive Cancer Center." Abstract. *Journal of Clinical Oncology* 37, 15, supplement (2019): 549. https://doi.org/10.1200/JCO.2019.37.15_suppl.549. https://ascopubs.org/doi/abs/10.1200/JCO.2019.37.15_suppl.549.

Lucas, Robyn M., and Rachael M. Rodney Harris. "On the Nature of Evidence and 'Proving' Causality: Smoking and Lung Cancer vs. Sun Exposure, Vitamin D and Multiple Sclerosis." *International Journal of Environmental Research and Public Health* 15, no. 8 (August 12, 2018): 1726. https://doi.org/10.3390/ijerph15081726. https://www.ncbi.nlm.nih.gov/pubmed/30103527.

Mandal, Ananya. "Darla Shine Joins Anti-vaccination Campaigners, Increases Threat of Measles Outbreak in the US." *News Medical,* February 15, 2019. https://www.news-medical.net/news/20190215/Darla-Shine-joins-anti-vac cination-campaigners-increases-threat-of-measles-outbreak-in-US.aspx.

Margolies, Laurie, and Shivani Chaudhry. "Pushing Anxiety as a Risk of Screening Mammography Is Benevolent Sexism and Bad for Women's Health Outcomes." *Clinical Imaging* 68 (December 2020): 166–68. https://doi.org/10.1016/j.clinimag.2020.05.034. https://www.ncbi.nlm.nih.gov/pubmed/32645603.

Martinez, Gina. "GoFundMe CEO: One-Third of Site's Donations Are to Cover Medical Costs." US, Healthcare. *Time,* updated January 30, 2019. https://time.com/5516037/gofundme-medical-bills-one-third-ceo/.

Mayo Clinic Breast Cancer Spore. "Measles Virus-Based Immunovirotherapy in the Treatment of Metastatic Breast Cancer." Mayo.edu, accessed June 17, 2021. https://www.mayo.edu/research/centers-programs/cancer-research/research-programs/womens-cancer-program/breast-cancer-spore/research -projects/measles-virus-based-immunovirotherapy-treatment-metastatic -breast-cancer.

Mayo Clinic staff. "Chemotherapy for Breast Cancer." MayoClinic.org, February 24, 2021. https://www.mayoclinic.org/tests-procedures/chemotherapy -for-breast-cancer/about/pac-20384931.

McCarthy, Sean L. "Jon Stewart Offers Rally to Restore Sanity Tips: Among Them, You Can Watch on Comedy Central or Online." *The Comic's Comic,* October 13, 2010. https://thecomicscomic.com/2010/10/13/jon-stewart -offers-rally-to-restore-sanity-tips-among-them-you-can-watch-on-comedy -central-or-online/.

Merlan, Anna. "The 'Energy Worker' Seen on Goop Has Implied that His Treatments Can Disappear Breast Cancer." Life. *Vice,* January 28, 2020. https://www.vice.com/en/article/939kk8/the-energy-worker-seen-on-goop -has-implied-that-his-treatments-can-disappear-breast-cancer.

McGreevey, Sue. "Why Antiangiogenesis Fails: Team Finds Possible Mechanism behind Resistance to Cancer Treatment." News and Research. Harvard Medical School, October 12, 2016. https://hms.harvard.edu/news/why-antiangiogenesis-fails.

Metastatic Breast Cancer Network. "Finding Financial Assistance." MBCN. org, accessed June 25, 2021. http://mbcn.org/finding-financial-assistance/.

Mohamed, Iftiin Hassan, Carmine Giorgio, Renato Bruni, Lisa Flammini, Elisabetta Barocelli, Damiano Rossi, Giuseppe Domenichini, Ferruccio Poli, and Massimiliano Tognolini. "Polyphenol Rich Botanicals Used as Food Supplements Interfere with EphA2-ephrinA1 System." *Pharmacologi-*

cal Research 64, no. 5 (November 2011): 464–70. https://doi.org/10.1016/j
.phrs.2011.06.008. https://www.ncbi.nlm.nih.gov/pubmed/21742039.

Mukherjee, Siddhartha. *The Emperor of All Maladies: A Biography of Cancer.*
New York: Scribner, 2010.

Musa, Julian, Marie-Ming Aynaud, Olivier Mirabeau, Olivier Delattre, and
Thomas G. P. Grünewald. "MYBL2 (B-Myb): A Central Regulator of Cell
Proliferation, Cell Survival and Differentiation Involved in Tumorigenesis."
Cell Death and Disease 8, no. 6 (June 22, 2017): e2895. https://doi.org/10.1038/
cddis.2017.244. https://www.ncbi.nlm.nih.gov/pubmed/28640249.

Nadler, Yasmine, A. M. González, Robert L. Camp, David L. Rimm, Harriet
M. Kluger, and Yuval Kluger. "Growth Factor Receptor-Bound Protein-7
(Grb7) as a Prognostic Marker and Therapeutic Target in Breast Cancer."
Annals of Oncology 21, no. 3 (March 2010): 466–73. https://doi.org/10.1093/
annonc/mdp346. https://www.ncbi.nlm.nih.gov/pubmed/19717535.

National Breast Cancer Foundation, Inc. "BRCA: The Breast Cancer Gene."
Last reviewed April 15, 2020. https://www.nationalbreastcancer.org/what
-is-brca.

———. "Breast Cancer Support Group." Accessed June 25, 2021. https://www
.nationalbreastcancer.org/nbcf-programs/breast-cancer-support-group.

———. "Mammography: Everything You Need to Know about Your Mammogram." Accessed June 18, 2021. https://www.nationalbreastcancer.org/
mammogram.

———. "Types." Last reviewed April 15, 2020. https://www.nationalbreastcan-
cer.org/types-of-breast-cancer/.

National Cancer Institute. "Basic and Translational Disparities Research
Funding." National Institutes of Health, Cancer.gov, updated January
13, 2021. https://www.cancer.gov/about-nci/organization/crchd/disparities
-research/basic-research.

———. "Cancer Stat Facts: Female Breast Cancer Subtypes." Surveillance,
Epidemiology, and End Results Program. Accessed June 25, 2021, https://
seer.cancer.gov/statfacts/html/breast-subtypes.html.

———. *Chemotherapy and You: Support for People with Cancer.* NIH publication
no. 18-7157. [Washington, DC]: US Department of Health and Human
Services and the National Cancer Institute Office of Communications and
Public Liaison, 2018. https://www.cancer.gov/publications/patient-educa
tion/chemotherapy-and-you.pdf.

———. "Clinical Trials Using Marijuana." National Institutes of Health,
Cancer.gov, accessed June 25, 2021. https://www.cancer.gov/about-cancer/
treatment/clinical-trials/intervention/marijuana.

———. "Metastasis: How Cancer Spreads." National Institutes of Health, US Department of Health and Human Services, December 2016. https://www.youtube.com/watch?v=fQwar_-QdiQ.

———. *Radiation Therapy and You: Support for People with Cancer*. NIH publication no. 17-7157. [Washington, DC]: US Department of Heath and Human Services and the National Institutes of Health, 2016. https://www.cancer.gov/publications/patient-education/radiationttherapy.pdf.

———. *What You Need to Know about Breast Cancer*. Booklet. NIH publication no. 12-1556. Revised August 2012. https://pubs.cancer.gov/pdf/Insides-wyntk-breast.pdf.

National Institutes of Health. "Cancer Disparities." National Cancer Institute, Cancer.gov, updated November 17, 2020. https://www.cancer.gov/about-cancer/understanding/disparities.

———. "Cannabis and Cannabinoids (PDQ®)–Health Professional Version." National Cancer Institute, Cancer.gov, updated June 3, 2021. https://www.cancer.gov/about-cancer/treatment/cam/hp/cannabis-pdq.

———. "Effects of Cannabis Use in Stage III–IV Non-small Cell Lung Cancer Patients." National Cancer Institute, Cancer.gov, accessed June 24, 2021. https://www.cancer.gov/about-cancer/treatment/clinical-trials/search/v?id=NCI-2020-01067&r=1.

———. "Hormones." National Cancer Institute, Cancer.gov, April 29, 2015. https://www.cancer.gov/about-cancer/causes-prevention/risk/hormones.

———. "Mammograms." National Cancer Institute, Cancer.gov, last reviewed December 7, 2016. https://www.cancer.gov/types/breast/mammograms-fact-sheet.

———. "Sentinel Lymph Node Biopsy." National Cancer Institute, Cancer.gov, reviewed June 25, 2019. https://www.cancer.gov/about-cancer/diagnosis-staging/staging/sentinel-node-biopsy-fact-sheet.

NCI staff. "Large Study Confirms that HPV Vaccine Prevents Cervical Cancer." National Institutes of Health, National Cancer Institute, Cancer.gov, October 14, 2020. https://www.cancer.gov/news-events/cancer-currents-blog/2020/hpv-vaccine-prevents-cervical-cancer-sweden-study.

Neuhouser, Marian L., Ashley Wilder Smith, Stephanie M. George, James T. Gibson, Kathy B. Baumgartner, Richard Baumgartner, Catherine Duggan, Leslie Bernstein, Anne McTiernan, and Rachel Ballard. "Use of Complementary and Alternative Medicine and Breast Cancer Survival in the Health, Eating, Activity, and Lifestyle Study." *Breast Cancer Research and Treatment* 160, no. 3 (December 2016): 539–46. https://doi.org/10.1007/s10549-016-4010-x. https://www.ncbi.nlm.nih.gov/pubmed/27766453.

Neuman, Heather, Jessica Schumacher, Bret Hanlon, Stephen Edge, Kathryn Ruddy, Ann Partridge, Jennifer Le-Rademacher, et al. "Local Recurrence Rates after Breast-Conserving Therapy in Patients Receiving Modern Era Therapy." American Society of Breast Surgeons, nineteenth annual meeting, Orlando, FL, May 4, 2018. See pp. 19–20 in https://www.breastsurgeons .org/docs/resources/old_meetings/2018_Official_Proceedings_ASBrS.pdf.

Neural Academy. "Cyclins and CDKs Cell Cycle Regulation." Video. YouTube, uploaded May 1, 2018. https://www.youtube.com/watch?v=nEMMKzYQf9A.

Newman, Lisa A., and Linda M. Kaljee. "Health Disparities and Triple-Negative Breast Cancer in African American Women: A Review." JAMA Surgery 152, no. 5 (May 1, 2017): 485–93. https://doi.org/10.1001/jama surg.2017.0005. https://www.ncbi.nlm.nih.gov/pubmed/28355428.

Ni, Chao, Liu Yang, Qiuran Xu, Hongjun Yuan, Wei Wang, Wenjie Xia, Dihe Gong, Wei Zhang, and Kun Yu. "CD68- and CD163-Positive Tumor Infiltrating Macrophages in Non-metastatic Breast Cancer: A Retrospective Study and Meta-Analysis." Journal of Cancer 10, no. 19 (2019): 4463–72. https://doi.org/10.7150/jca.33914. https://www.ncbi.nlm.nih.gov/ pubmed/31528210.

Nicolini, Andrea, Paola Ferrari, and Michael J. Duffy. "Prognostic and Predictive Biomarkers in Breast Cancer: Past, Present and Future." Seminars in Cancer Biology 52, part 1 (October 2018): 56–73. https://doi.org/10.1016/j .semcancer.2017.08.010. https://www.ncbi.nlm.nih.gov/pubmed/28882552.

Notaro, Tig. Boyish Girl Interrupted. Album. Bentzen Ball Records and Secretly Canadian (label). Released August 5, 2016. https://www.hbo.com/specials/ tig-notaro-boyish-girl-interrupted/synopsis.

———. Live. Album. Pig Newton (label). Released October 5, 2012.

Obama, Michelle. Becoming. New York: Crown, 2018.

Odes, Edward J., Patrick S. Randolph-Quinney, Maryna Steyn, Zach Throckmorton, Jaqueline S. Smilg, Bernhard Zipfel, Tanya N. Augustine, et al. "Earliest Hominin Cancer: 1.7-Million-Year-Old Osteosarcoma from Swartkrans Cave, South Africa." Research article. South African Journal of Science 112, nos. 7/8 (2016): 1–5. https://doi.org/https://doi.org/10.17159/ sajs.2016/20150471. http://www.scielo.org.za/scielo.php?pid=S0038 -23532016000400014&script=sci_arttext&tlng=es.

Office of Infectious Diseases and HIV/AIDS Policy. "Vaccine Types." HHS. gov, Vaccines.gov, April 29, 2021. https://www.vaccines.gov/basics/types.

Oswalt, Patton. Patton Oswalt: Annihilation. Netflix. Released October 17, 2017. https://www.netflix.com/title/80177406.

Owens, Deirdre Cooper. Medical Bondage: Race, Gender, and the Origins of American Gynecology. Athens: University of Georgia Press, 2018.

Pahuja, Monica. "Breast Ultrasound." Breast Imaging. Inside Radiology (website), last modified August 13, 2018. https://www.insideradiology.com.au/breast-ultrasound/.

Papadakis, Emmanouil S., Thomas Reeves, Natalia H. Robson, Tom Maishman, Graham Packham, and Ramsey I. Cutress. "BAG-1 as a Biomarker in Early Breast Cancer Prognosis: A Systematic Review with Meta-Analyses." *British Journal of Cancer* 116, no. 12 (June 6, 2017): 1585–94. https://doi.org/10.1038/bjc.2017.130. https://www.ncbi.nlm.nih.gov/pubmed/28510570.

Parsons, Faith. "Myc Gene Faith Parsons." Video. YouTube, uploaded January 22, 2019. https://www.youtube.com/watch?v=e3tN-WVUSa8.

Patient Advocate Foundation. "Breast Cancer Resource Directory." Accessed June 25, 2021. https://www.patientadvocate.org/explore-our-resources/breast-cancer-resource-directory/.

PDQ® Integrative, Alternative, and Complementary Therapies Editorial Board. *PDQ Cannabis and Cannabinoids.* Bethesda, MD: National Cancer Institute, updated June 3, 2021. https://www.cancer.gov/about-cancer/treatment/cam/hp/cannabis-pdq.

Penner, Louis A., John F. Dovidio, Nao Hagiwara, Tanina Foster, Terrance L. Albrecht, Robert A. Chapman, and Susan Eggly. "An Analysis of Race-Related Attitudes and Beliefs in Black Cancer Patients: Implications for Health Care Disparities." *Journal of Health Care for the Poor and Underserved* 27, no. 3 (2016): 1503–20. https://doi.org/10.1353/hpu.2016.0115. https://www.ncbi.nlm.nih.gov/pubmed/27524781.

Pratt-Chapman, Mandi L., and Jennifer Potter. *Cancer Care Considerations for Sexual and Gender Minority Patients.* [Rockville, MD]: Association of Community Cancer Centers, 2019. https://www.accc-cancer.org/docs/documents/oncology-issues/articles/nd19/nd19-cancer-care-considerations-for-sexual-and-gender-minority-patients.pdf.

Pressley, Sue Ann. "Hate May Have Triggered Fatal Barracks Beating." *Washington Post,* August 11, 1999. https://www.washingtonpost.com/wp-srv/national/daily/aug99/winchell11.htm.

RadiologyInfo.org. "Mammography." Reviewed April 12, 2019. https://www.radiologyinfo.org/en/info.cfm?pg=mammo.

Reuben, Suzanne H., Erin L. Milliken, and Lisa J. Paradis. *The Future of Cancer Research: Accelerating Scientific Innovation.* President's Cancer Panel Annual Report, 2010–2011. [Bethesda, MD]: US Department of Health and Human Services and the National Institutes of Health, 2012. https://deainfo.nci.nih.gov/advisory/pcp/annualreports/pcp10-11rpt/FullReport.pdf.

Ridley, Jim. "Losing the Connection." *Nashville Scene*, March 17, 2005. https:// www.nashvillescene.com/news/article/13011506/losing-the-connection.

RIKEN Omics Science Center. "The Central Dogma: From Genomic Information to Protein Synthesis." Video. Made as part of the Beyond Genetics exhibit at the National Science Museum of Japan. 2007. https://www.youtube .com/watch?v=-ygpqVr7_xs.

Rowshanravan, Behzad, Neil Halliday, and David M. Sansom. "CTLA-4: A Moving Target in Immunotherapy." *Blood* 131, no. 1 (January 4, 2018): 58–67. https://doi.org/10.1182/blood-2017-06-741033. https://www.ncbi .nlm.nih.gov/pubmed/29118008.

Rudzińska, Magdalena, Alessandro Parodi, Surinder M. Soond, Andrey Z. Vinarov, Dmitry O. Korolev, Andrey O. Morozov, Cenk Daglioglu, Yusuf Tutar, and Andrey A. Zamyatnin Jr. "The Role of Cysteine Cathepsins in Cancer Progression and Drug Resistance." *International Journal of Molecular Sciences* 20, no. 14 (July 23, 2019): 3602. https://doi.org/10.3390/ijms20143602. https://www.ncbi.nlm.nih.gov/pubmed/31340550.

Russell, Stephen J., Dusica Babovic-Vuksanovic, Alice Bexon, Roberto Cattaneo, David Dingli, Angela Dispenzieri, David R. Deyle, et al. "Oncolytic Measles Virotherapy and Opposition to Measles Vaccination." *Mayo Clinic Proceedings* 94, no. 9 (2019): 1834–39. https://doi.org/https://doi .org/10.1016/j.mayocp.2019.05.006. https://www.mayoclinicproceedings .org/article/S0025-6196(19)30462-8/pdf.

Sabin, Janice A. "How We Fail Black Patients in Pain." Insights. *Association of American Medical Colleges News*, January 6, 2020. https://www.aamc.org/ news-insights/how-we-fail-black-patients-pain.

Sacks, Tina K. *Invisible Visits: Black Middle-Class Women in the American Healthcare System*. Oxford: Oxford University Press, 2019.

Scharff, Darcell P., Katherine J. Mathews, Pamela Jackson, Jonathan Hoffsuemmer, Emeobong Martin, and Dorothy Edwards. "More than Tuskegee: Understanding Mistrust about Research Participation." *Journal of Health Care for the Poor and Underserved* 21, no. 3 (August 2010): 879–97. https://doi .org/10.1353/hpu.0.0323. https://www.ncbi.nlm.nih.gov/pubmed/20693733.

SciShow. "Why We Haven't Cured Cancer." Video. Uploaded May 14, 2015. https://www.youtube.com/watch?v=7tzaWOdvGMw.

Sealy, Andy. "'If Ya Don't Know, Now Ya Know': A Guide to What Is Needed Post-mastectomy." *Focus on Cancer Blog*, Penn Medicine, Abramson Cancer Center, October 23, 2018. https://www.pennmedicine.org/cancer/about/ focus-on-cancer/2018/october/list-of-post-mastectomy-items-needed.

Seto, Belinda. "Rapamycin and mTOR: A Serendipitous Discovery and Implications for Breast Cancer." *Clinical and Translational Medicine* 1, no. 1

(November 15, 2012): e29. https://doi.org/10.1186/2001-1326-1-29. https:// www.ncbi.nlm.nih.gov/pubmed/23369283.

Sharpless, Norman E. "Funding from Congress Allows NCI to Raise Grants Payline." National Institutes of Health, National Cancer Institute, Cancer. gov, February 4, 2021. https://www.cancer.gov/grants-training/nci-bottom -line-blog/2021/funding-from-congress-allows-nci-to-raise-grants-payline.

Shi, Siyu, Arthur R. Brant, Aaron Sabolch, and Erqi Pollom. "False News of a Cannabis Cancer Cure." Cureus 11, no. 1 (January 19, 2019): e3918. https://doi.org/10.7759/cureus.3918. https://www.ncbi.nlm.nih.gov/ pubmed/30931189.

Sirugo, Giorgio, Scott M. Williams, and Sarah A. Tishkoff. "The Missing Diversity in Human Genetic Studies." Cell 177, no. 4 (May 2, 2019): 1080. https://doi.org/10.1016/j.cell.2019.04.032. https://pubmed.ncbi.nlm .nih.gov/31051100/.

Skloot, Rebecca. The Immortal Life of Henrietta Lacks. New York: Crown Publishing Group, 2010.

Smithsonian National Museum of American History. "The Iron Lung and Other Equipment," Whatever Happened to Polio? Accessed June 17, 2021. https://amhistory.si.edu/polio/howpolio/ironlung.htm.

Song, Wenqiang, Yoonha Hwang, Victoria M. Youngblood, Rebecca S. Cook, Justin M. Balko, Jin Chen, and Dana M. Brantley-Sieders. "Targeting EphA2 Impairs Cell Cycle Progression and Growth of Basal-like/ Triple-Negative Breast Cancers." Oncogene 36, no. 40 (October 5, 2017): 5620–30. https://doi.org/10.1038/onc.2017.170. https://www.ncbi.nlm.nih. gov/pubmed/28581527.

Speaking of Research. "Medical Benefits." Accessed June 18, 2021. https:// speakingofresearch.com/facts/medical-benefits/.

Stanborough, Rebecca Joy. "What Are Cognitive Distortions and How Can You Change These Thinking Patterns? 'Should' Statements." Healthline, December 18, 2019. https://www.healthline.com/health/cognitive -distortions#should-statements.

Steele, C. Brooke, Julie S. Townsend, Elizabeth A. Courtney-Long, and Monique Young. "Prevalence of Cancer Screening among Adults with Disabilities, United States, 2013." Preventing Chronic Disease 14 (January 26, 2017): E09. https://doi.org/10.5888/pcd14.160312. https://www.ncbi.nlm .nih.gov/pubmed/28125399.

Strait, Julia Evangelou. "Breast Cancer Vaccine Shows Promise in Small Clinical Trial." Siteman Cancer Center, Washington University School of Medicine, accessed June 17, 2021. https://siteman.wustl.edu/breast-cancer -vaccine-shows-promise-in-small-clinical-trial/.

Strenger, Rochelle, Howard Safran, and Cooper Woodward. "Autism and Cancer: Creating Comprehensive Solutions for Complex Needs." *ASCO Daily News*, January 3, 2020. https://dailynews.ascopubs.org/do/10.1200/ADN.19.190488/full/.

Sun, Xiaoming, and Paul D. Kaufman. "Ki-67: More than a Proliferation Marker." *Chromosoma* 127, no. 2 (June 2018): 175–86. https://doi.org/10.1007/s00412-018-0659-8. https://www.ncbi.nlm.nih.gov/pubmed/29322240.

Susan G. Komen. "Lumpectomy: The Procedure." Komen.org, updated May 18, 2021. https://www.komen.org/breast-cancer/treatment/type/surgery/lumpectomy/procedure-information/.

———. "Survival and Risk of Recurrence after Treatment." Komen.org, updated May 24, 2021. https://www.komen.org/breast-cancer/survivorship/medical-care/survival-and-risk-of-recurrence/.

———. "Susan G. Komen Treatment Assistance Program." Komen.org, August 2020. https://www.komen.org/wp-content/uploads/2020-Komen-TAP-Helpline-Flyer-Eng-Aug-2.pdf.

Sykes, Wanda. *Wanda Sykes: Not Normal*. Netflix. Released May 21, 2019. https://www.netflix.com/title/81011598.

Tang, Weifeng, Hao Qiu, Heping Jiang, Lixin Wang, Bin Sun, and Haiyong Gu. "Aurora-A V57I (rs1047972) Polymorphism and Cancer Susceptibility: A Meta-Analysis Involving 27,269 Subjects." *PLoS One* 9, no. 3 (2014): e90328. https://doi.org/10.1371/journal.pone.0090328. https://www.ncbi.nlm.nih.gov/pubmed/24598702.

Tein, Caroline. "FDA Clears Breast Cancer Vaccine for Clinical Trials." Health News. *Verywell Health*, January 8, 2021. https://www.verywellhealth.com/breast-cancer-vaccine-greenlit-clinical-trials-5094403.

Tian, Sun, Paul Roepman, Laura J. Van't Veer, Rene Bernards, Femke de Snoo, and Annuska M. Glas. "Biological Functions of the Genes in the MammaPrint Breast Cancer Profile Reflect the Hallmarks of Cancer." *Biomarker Insights* 5 (November 28, 2010): 129–38. https://doi.org/10.4137/BMI.S6184. https://www.ncbi.nlm.nih.gov/pubmed/21151591.

Tian, Yonggui, Yilu Li, Yupei Shao, and Yi Zhang. "Gene Modification Strategies for Next-Generation CAR T Cells against Solid Cancers." *Journal of Hematology and Oncology* 13, no. 1 (May 18, 2020): 54. https://doi.org/10.1186/s13045-020-00890-6. https://pubmed.ncbi.nlm.nih.gov/32423475/.

US Department of Defense. "Program Announcement for the Department of Defense, Defense Health Program, Congressionally Directed Medical Research Programs, Breast Cancer Research Program Breakthrough Award

Levels 1 and 2." CDMRP (website), accessed June 17, 2021. https://cdmrp .army.mil/funding/pa/fy19-bcrp-bta12.pdf.

US Food and Drug Administration. "FDA News Release: FDA Approves New Therapy for Triple Negative Breast Cancer that Has Spread, Not Responded to Other Treatments." News release. FDA.gov, April 22, 2020. https:// www.fda.gov/news-events/press-announcements/fda-approves-new-therapy -triple-negative-breast-cancer-has-spread-not-responded-other-treatments.

———. "Lupron Depot® 7.5 Mg (Leuprolide Acetate for Depot Suspension)." Drug information sheet. FDA.gov, October 7, 2011. https://www.accessdata .fda.gov/drugsatfda_docs/label/2012/019732s038lbl.pdf.

US National Library of Medicine. "Evaluation of Lasofoxifene versus Fulves-trant in Advanced or Metastatic ER+/HER2– Breast Cancer with an ESR1 Mutation." ClinicalTrials.gov, National Institutes of Health, accessed June 18, 2021. https://clinicaltrials.gov/ct2/show/NCT03781063.

———. "Study BT5528-100 in Patients with Advanced Solid Tumors As-sociated with EphA2 Expression." ClinicalTrials.gov, National Institutes of Health, accessed June 24, 2021. https://clinicaltrials.gov/ct2/show/ NCT04180371.

University of Iowa Health Care. "Study Discovers Link berween Cancer and Autism: Patients with Autism Have Increased Gene Mutations that Drive Cancer, but Lower Rates of Cancer." ScienceDaily, April 13, 2016. https:// www.sciencedaily.com/releases/2016/04/160413120954.htm.

University of Washington Family Medicine. "Everything Is Awful and I'm Not Okay: Questions to Ask before Giving Up." 2015. https://depts.washington .edu/fammed/wp-content/uploads/2019/03/Katers-selfcare_printable.pdf.

University of Wisconsin Population Health Institute. "Cultural Competence Training for Health Care Professionals." County Health Rankings (web-site), last updated January 17, 2020. https://www.countyhealthrankings.org/ take-action-to-improve-health/what-works-for-health/strategies/cultural -competence-training-for-health-care-professionals.

Vanderbilt University Medical Center. "A New National Study Will Assess Microsurgery Reinnervation." Discover, July 3, 2019. https://discover.vumc .org/2019/07/resensation-after-breast-reconstruction/.

———. "Vanderbilt Surgeons Lead Nation in Study to Restore Sensation in Breast Tissue." VUMC Reporter, May 23, 2019. https://news.vumc .org/2019/05/23/vanderbilt-surgeons-lead-nation-in-study-to-restore-sensa tion-in-breast-tissue/.

Vaught, David B., Alyssa R. Merkel, Conor C. Lynch, James Edwards, Mo-hammed Noor Tantawy, Timothy Hilliard, Shan Wang, Todd Peterson, Rachelle W. Johnson, Julie A. Sterling, and Dana Brantley-Sieders. "EphA2

Is a Clinically Relevant Target for Breast Cancer Bone Metastatic Disease." *JBMR Plus* 5, no. 4 (April 2021): e10465. https://doi.org/10.1002/jbm4.10465, https://pubmed.ncbi.nlm.nih.gov/33869989/.

Wang, Amy B. "Gwyneth Paltrow's Goop Touted the 'Benefits' of Putting a Jade Egg in Your Vagina. Now It Must Pay." *Washington Post*, September 5, 2018. https://www.washingtonpost.com/health/2018/09/05/gwyneth-paltrows-goop-touted-benefits-putting-jade-egg-your-vagina-now-it-must-pay/.

Wang, Jiani, and Binghe Xu. "Targeted Therapeutic Options and Future Perspectives for HER2-Positive Breast Cancer." *Signal Transduct and Targeted Therapy* 4 (September 13, 2019): 34. https://doi.org/10.1038/s41392-019-0069-2. https://www.ncbi.nlm.nih.gov/pubmed/31637013.

WebMD. "HER2+ Breast Cancer Survival Rates." Breast Cancer Guide. Last reviewed May 17, 2020. https://www.webmd.com/breast-cancer/guide/her2-positive-breast-cancer-survival-rates.

Wolfe, David. "Medicinal Mushroom Benefits: What Does the Science Have to Say?" DavidWolfe.com, June 3, 2019. https://shop.davidwolfe.com/blogs/health/medicinal-mushrooms.

———. "Vitamin B17 May Treat Cancer, but Is Illegal in the US!" DavidWolfe.com, accessed June 17, 2021. https://www.davidwolfe.com/vitamin-b17-kills-cancer-illegal-us/.

Wright, Jessica. "Dozens of Autism Genes Have Cancer Connections." *Spectrum News*, June 10, 2016. https://www.spectrumnews.org/news/dozens-of-autism-genes-have-cancer-connections/.

Yabroff, K. Robin, Katherine Reeder-Hayes, Jingxuan Zhao, Michael T. Halpern, Ana Maria Lopez, Leon Bernal-Mizrachi, Anderson B. Collier, et al. "Health Insurance Coverage Disruptions and Cancer Care and Outcomes: Systematic Review of Published Research." *Journal of the National Cancer Institute* 112, no. 7 (July 1, 2020): 671–87. https://doi.org/10.1093/jnci/djaa048. https://www.ncbi.nlm.nih.gov/pubmed/32337585.

Yabroff, K. Robin, Ted Gansler, Richard C. Wender, Kevin J. Cullen, and Otis W. Brawley. "Minimizing the Burden of Cancer in the United States: Goals for a High-Performing Health Care System." *CA: A Cancer Journal for Clinicians* 69, no. 3 (May/June 2019): 166–83. https://doi.org/10.3322/caac.21556. https://www.ncbi.nlm.nih.gov/pubmed/30786025.

YaleCourse. "Cancer as an Evolutionary Process: Clonal Evolution." Video. Uploaded May 14, 2014. https://www.youtube.com/watch?v=wH9jmQglOLw.

Ye, Chenyang, Ji Wang, Pin Wu, Xiaofen Li, and Ying Chai. "Prognostic Role of Cyclin B1 in Solid Tumors: A Meta-Analysis." *Oncotarget* 8, no. 2 (January 10, 2017): 2224–32. https://doi.org/10.18632/oncotarget.13653. https://www.ncbi.nlm.nih.gov/pubmed/27903976.

Yip, Cheng-Har, and Anthony Rhodes. "Estrogen and Progesterone Receptors in Breast Cancer." *Future Oncology* 10, no. 14 (November 2014): 2293–2301. https://doi.org/10.2217/fon.14.110. https://www.ncbi.nlm.nih .gov/pubmed/25471040.

Yuko, Elizabeth. "How to Avoid Toxic Positivity (And Handle It When It Comes Your Way)." *Lifehacker*, September 6, 2020. https://lifehacker.com/ how-to-avoid-toxic-positivity-and-handle-it-when-it-co-1844966691.

Zavala, Valentina A., Paige M. Bracci, John M. Carethers, Luis Carvajal-Carmona, Nicole B. Coggins, Marcia R. Cruz-Correa, Melissa Davis, et al. "Cancer Health Disparities in Racial/Ethnic Minorities in the United States." *British Journal of Cancer* 124, no. 2 (January 2021): 315–32. https://doi.org/10.1038/s41416-020-01038-6. https://www.ncbi.nlm.nih .gov/pubmed/32901135.

Zhang, Cheng, Jun Liu, Jiang F. Zhong, and Xi Zhang. "Engineering CAR-T Cells." *Biomarker Research* 5 (June 24, 2017): 22. https://doi.org/10.1186/ s40364-017-0102-y. https://www.ncbi.nlm.nih.gov/pubmed/28652918.

Zhang, Jian, Ying Wu, Xichun Hu, Biyun Wang, Leiping Wang, Sheng Zhang, Jun Cao, and Zhonghua Wang. "GSTT1, GSTP1, and GSTM1 Genetic Variants Are Associated with Survival in Previously Untreated Metastatic Breast Cancer." *Oncotarget* 8, no. 62 (December 1, 2017): 105905–14. https://doi.org/10.18632/oncotarget.22450. https://www.ncbi.nlm.nih.gov/ pubmed/29285301.

Index

About the Author

Dr. **Dana M. Brantley-Sieders** is an academic researcher who has worked at Vanderbilt University Medical Center for twenty years and counting. She studies molecular mechanisms that regulate breast-tumor cell growth, angiogenesis, and metastatic spread, working to identify new drug targets and to target conventionally undruggable targets with nanoparticle- and nanocarrier-delivered siRNA. Over her career, she's contributed to more than fifty peer-reviewed studies. She has worked with Susan G. Komen for the Cure's Central Tennessee Affiliate to identify and target resource allocation over the affiliate area to meet the diverse needs of rural and urban populations, and she regularly volunteers her time to local schools, speaking about science. Since her diagnosis with breast cancer in 2018, she has become an advocate for breast cancer patients and survivors as well as an advocate for science. On her blog, talkingtatas.com, she regularly covers breast cancer, cancer biology, scientific advances in the field of breast cancer, and beyond, shares personal stories, and debunks pseudoscience scams. In addition to maintaining a career in biomedical research, she's the mother of two children and three fur-children and spends her spare time writing fiction under the name D. B. Sieders, gardening, and flying with her personal pilot/husband.